UNMASKING ADDICTION!

EXPLORING THE DEPTHS OF OBSESSIONS AND PASSIONS: A HOLISTIC APPROACH TO UNDERSTANDING AND HEALING!

PIERRE J. SAMAAN, PH.D.

WESTBOW
PRESS®
A DIVISION OF THOMAS NELSON
& ZONDERVAN

WestBow Press books may be ordered through booksellers or by contacting:

WestBow Press
A Division of Thomas Nelson & Zondervan
1663 Liberty Drive
Bloomington, IN 47403
www.westbowpress.com
844-714-3454

ISBN: 979-8-3850-2624-1 (sc)
ISBN: 979-8-3850-2625-8 (e)

Library of Congress Control Number: 2024910687

Print information available on the last page.

WestBow Press rev. date: 06/17/2024

CONTENTS

CHAPTER 1

INTRODUCTION

Addiction has many meanings. Too many people express nothing good about the subject. Perhaps synonyms best describe addiction as an obsession with, infatuation with, passion for, love for, fondness for, a weakness for, penchant for, a propensity for, appetite for, or mania for.[1]

Alcoholics Anonymous gives the most popular definition of addiction as "an inability to stop using a substance or engaging in a behavior even though it is causing psychological and physical harm." The AA Introductory Pamphlet describes the addiction to alcoholism as "A physical compulsion, coupled with a mental obsession."[2]

Our focus on addiction is not solely on one use or user. We are attempting to understand better compulsive behavior attached to obsessive thinking as a spiritual "fact or condition of being addicted to a particular substance, thing, or activity."[3]

Today's most common addictions are alcohol, illicit substances/drugs, sex, internet, gambling, gaming, cell phones, work, and others.

Those with addiction issues wear a mask of normalcy for all to see. When looking into the mirror, they also desire to see the covering—mask—to hide what is underneath.

---

[1] Retrieved from https://www.lexico.com/synonyms/addiction
[2] https://www.aa.org/sites/default/files/literature/assets/p-1_thisisaa1.pdf
[3] https://www.medicalnewstoday.com/articles/323465#addiction-vs-misuse

Ritual masks can be very revealing when used to represent the human face. They disclose two fundamental aspects of the human condition: first, the hiding of the fear and apprehension-driven part of the self or soul (Limbic System—Brain's basement); second, the self-protective, egocentric intellect that turns selfishly angry when threatened or exposed—often seen as hypocrisy.

The title "Unmasking Addiction" reveals a condition that can quickly destroy a person's spirit, soul, and body. Not only does this condition damage the thinking and emotional faculties of the mind/soul, but it also sets into motion an interplay of impairing physiological functioning that ravages the body.

The consequential loss of the human spirit and identity places God in the background. "Look at yourself," addiction tells its victim. "God doesn't want an addict. You're not good enough. You're not ready. There will be time for that later."

Of course, later never comes because addictive thinking has taken over. *Emotional reasoning (I feel good, so this must be good!)* is now in control. And the addictive process, which may have begun innocently enough, becomes a monster from within—a beast with the lure of a seductress entrapping its victim into a dichotomy of desire and pain.

In "Unmasking Addiction" we identify six essential areas involving spirit, soul, and body addiction. These six areas are:

1. Unmasking Spiritual Origins of the Addictive Process
2. Unmasking Behavioral Origins of the Addictive Process
3. Unmasking the Addictive Personality
4. Unmasking Drugs and the Brain
5. Unmasking Recovery
6. Unmasking Relapse

"Some say: 'I am free to do everything'—but not everything is healthy. I am free to do everything, but I will not do anything that destroys my autonomy and takes away my freedom." (1 Corinthians 6:12 REM)

SPIRITUAL ORIGINS OF THE ADDICTIVE PROCESS

In removing the covering of addiction, what will we find? Is addiction being controlled by something because you need it? Or is addiction a way of life, self-medication, self-soothing, a moral weakness, a mental illness, a disease, an allergy, a spiritual sickness (sin), or a genetic, environmental, or drug-induced disorder?

Someone asked if we could find illustrations of addiction in the Bible. The answer is that there are innumerable examples of addiction in written Bible stories.

Of course, the first mention of alcohol use and abuse was with Noah (Genesis 9:18-23). However, Noah was a man of God, known to have good character, and diligently served God while building the ark.

Within an agricultural growing season after the waters covering the earth subsided. After the flood, Noah indulged himself in intoxication after harvesting his first crop of grapes from the new rich soil. However, in Noah's history, no typical addiction character traits indicate an alcoholic.

Nabal's Story!

One Bible story that immediately comes to mind is that of Nabal, whose offense triggered David into an evil, murderous plan.

Nabal is a different example from Noah as someone who became intoxicated in the Bible. In 1 Samuel 25:1-44, we read how Nabal's alcoholism became his downfall.

The story of Nabal describes a man of the opposite character to Noah. We can summarize Nabal's character traits as among the lowest personalities. Not even his wife, Abigail, had a good word to say about Nabal, calling him *"a wicked man. . .his name means Fool and folly goes with him. . ."* (vs. 25)

Nabal's servants named him among one of the "sons of Belial," meaning sons of Satan and sons of worthlessness. The name Belial is a derivative of the demon "Belil" (without the "a"), one of the original fallen angels.

Nabal's Character of Addiction

Nabal's unflattering character is that of a **"harsh"** (vs. 10, 11, 17) man who is unpleasantly rough and cruel to everyone. He is known to be egocentrically **"selfish"** (v. 11), disregarding others, including his wife. Nabal spoke with **"arrogance"** (v. 9) to David's men and everyone else. **"Rageful"** (v. 14), Nabal was prone to cause others to sin, seeking revenge against him. Others consider him to be **"good for nothing"** (v. 17). He displayed a lack of self-control in **"drunkenness"** (v. 36). And his personality is observed by many in addiction. As seen by Abigail's fear of telling Nabal during his drunkenness about what she did to halt David's murderous intentions, Nabal was prone to unsafe behavior.

"When Abigail got home, she found Nabal presiding over a huge banquet. He was in high spirits—and very, very drunk. So she didn't tell him anything of what she'd done until morning." (1 Samuel 25:36 MSG)

I can't tell you the number of times I have heard wives expressing fears of communicating with their husbands acting out in their addiction — substance or behavioral addictions.

Is Addiction Considered A Curse?

When we look at the descriptions of Biblical curses, we see an expected result: either repentance and the curse lifting, or "being cursed includes loss of everything significant and a lowering to the most menial of positions."[4]

Does that sound like the results of most addictions? In Deuteronomy 27:15-26, we can see behaviors that could lead to being perceived as curses. Severe addictive behavior displays many of these maladaptive behaviors.

- Idolatry
- Incest
- Misleading the blind (or naive)

---

[4] Elwell, Walter A., Edit., Evangelical Dictionary of Biblical Theology. p. 139, Baker Book House Publishing, Grand Rapids, MI. 1996

- Ambush
- Disrespect for authority
- Subversion of justice

The most graphic scriptural depiction of a curse is given in Deuteronomy 28:16-68 when it describes the consequences that often occur upon the curse.

- Incurable diseases
- Slow starvation
- Abuse by enemies
- Exile
- Panic
- Confusion
- Madness

In the New Testament (Elwell, 1996, p. 139), "A curse came to mean total removal of a person from the company of the redeemed where all blessings are localized. Thus, *anathema* in the New Testament became equivalent to *herem* in the Old Testament. This curse was imposed for apostasy (Galatians 1:8), not loving Christ (1 Corinthians 16:22), and not extending loving care to the least of the brethren (Matthew 25:41)."[5]

You decide if the Bible is describing addiction as a curse. Ask yourself if you are going to an extreme with sports, work, shopping, substances, gambling, sex, relationships, or even family and children.

One thing is for sure. No matter what terrible condition we find ourselves in, God will never give up on us. God does not want us to be obsessed with anything other than Himself.

"For there is no temptation to discontinue God's treatment that has come upon you except for the fear and selfishness that infects all mankind. God is reliable and trustworthy; he will not allow temptation beyond your ability to resist, but when you are tempted, he will always provide resources, options, opportunities, support, and alternate ways out so that you can stand

---

[5] Ibid.

your ground and overcome the temptation, thereby growing stronger with each victory." (1 Corinthians 10:13 REM)

UNMASKING THE BEHAVIORAL ORIGINS OF THE ADDICTIVE PROCESS

Behavior is how one acts or conducts oneself in response to a particular situation or stimulus. Behavior is the response or reaction to events, thinking, and emotions, "The Think—Feel—Do Cycle."

Many will say that, unlike animals, human behavior is not instinctual — an inborn, typically fixed pattern of behavior, such as birds migrating south just before winter. Some have stretched the definition of instinct to include a sense or intuition more closely associated with the biblical human spirit rather than physiological attributes (brain/body) evoking behavior.

Others say humans have three primary survival instincts: Self-Preservation, Sexual, and Social. The three instinctual drives are promulgated by those who desire to prove the "true self" is derived from ancient sources from within, e.g., spirit beings, reincarnation, etc. Unfortunately, their historical claims have been proven to be false.[6]

Science-driven Human development, or Developmental Psychology, is a field of study that attempts to describe and explain the changes in human cognitive, emotional, and behavioral capabilities and functioning over the entire life span, from embryonic conception to old age.[7] Addiction is rooted in **human development**, the growth and change process between conception and maturity.

The addictive person is the offshoot of human development, from the origins of our DNA to the environmental interactions crafting character development. In other words, addictive behavior is an offshoot of genes & decisions.

We are <u>not</u> born to be an addict! Yes, we may have a DNA sequence

---

[6] Retrieved from file:///Users/pierresamaan/Documents/My%20Files/BIBLE/Enneagram_Decoding%20the%20Origins%20of%20the%20Enneagram%20—%20Cultish.webarchive

[7] Retrieved from https://www.britannica.com/topic/human-behavior

that predisposes specific characteristics. However, we emphasize or subjugate healthy and unhealthy traits — inclinations.

One can regard an inclination as bias leading to a habit developed by choice within self-control and possessing the means or skills to break the pattern at any time.

Conversely, many define an addictive person as being out of control with a belief, emotion, or behavior (substance, gambling, sex, etc.); psychological and physical components of the "Think—Feel—Do Cycle" on steroids. Is the addict in or out of control; "I didn't mean to do it!"

Addiction's behavioral origins or causes are a combination of emotional, mental, and physical factors (spirit, soul, body) within an addict's life span.

The Bible Says...

"For everything in the world (including sinful people) is infected with selfishness, and this selfishness is expressed in three primary avenues: sensualism, materialism, and egotism. And this terminal infection does not come from the Father but is part of this sick world. This sick world and its selfish desires will pass away, but those who willingly experience God's healing and re-creation of hearts and minds will live forever."
(1 John 2:16 REM)

CHAPTER 2

FAMILY SYSTEM — "DYSFUNCTIONAL FAMILY SYSTEM OF ADDICTION'S BEHAVIORAL ORIGIN!"

An impaired family system consists of negative family dynamics, which are harmful or destructive patterns of interaction between family members instead of supportive and constructive ones. The dysfunctional family system encompasses issues such as dysfunctional communication, enmeshment, triangulation, parentification, and neglect & abuse. These dynamics can heavily impact family members' mental, emotional, spiritual, and, at times, physical well-being. Now, let us explore the potential effects of these typical negative family dynamics.

A predominant characteristic is *dysfunctional communication*. This involves a need for more open and honest communication within the family. Researchers have identified communication patterns that predict the success or failure of relationships, including familial ones.

Family members may resort to passive-aggressive behavior, avoid discussing important issues, or use sarcasm and criticism rather than expressing themselves clearly and respectfully (Gottman 1994).[8]

A typical characteristic of a dysfunctional family system is *enmeshment*. In an enmeshed family, boundaries between members are

---

[8] Gottman, J. M. (1994). "Why Marriages Succeed or Fail: And How You Can Make Yours Last". Simon & Schuster.

weak or nonexistent. Members may need more personal space and an inability to develop independently. This can lead to over-dependence on family approval and difficulty forming outside relationships (Minuchin 1974).[9] This dynamic can lead to anxiety, depression, and addictive behaviors to escape coping with stress due to the lack of personal autonomy and over-reliance on family.

Triangulation occurs when two family members, instead of dealing with their conflict directly, bring in a third member to mediate or take sides. This dynamic can create alliances and splits within the family, fostering misunderstanding and resentment (Bowman 1978).[10]

Allow me to introduce you to the parents of the Anderson family, along with their two children, Mark and Lisa, and their 15-year-old daughter, Sophia. Mark and Lisa frequently find themselves at odds regarding financial matters within the family dynamic. Instead of directly resolving these conflicts, they involve Sophia in their communication. Whenever a disagreement arises between Mark and Lisa, rather than discussing it face-to-face, one of them will often confide in Sophia, entrusting her to relay messages to the other parent. Consequently, Sophia finds herself in a challenging position where she feels accountable for managing her parents' emotions and minimizing conflict. For instance, Lisa may vent her frustrations about Mark to Sophia, expecting empathy and support. Rather than addressing their marital issues head-on, the parents rely on Sophia to act as a mediator, placing an undue emotional burden on her shoulders.

One family member is unfairly blamed for problems within the family. This person, often a child, becomes the 'scapegoat' and is subjected to undue criticism and hostility, affecting their self-esteem and mental health (Akhtar 2019).[11]

From a Clinical Pastoral Counseling perspective, principles such as truthfulness, direct communication, and avoiding deceit and manipulation (Proverbs 12:22, Ephesians 4:25) are foundational. Counseling might

---

[9] Minuchin, S. (1974). "Families and Family Therapy". Harvard University Press.
[10] Bowen, M. (1978). "Family Therapy in Clinical Practice". Jason Aronson.
[11] Akhtar, S. (Ed.). (2019). "The Scapegoat Complex: Toward a Mythology of Shadow and Guilt". Routledge.

encourage family members to communicate openly and honestly with each other, fostering an environment of trust and healing.

Parentification is a role reversal where a child is placed in an adult role, taking on responsibilities and emotional burdens typically associated with a parent. This dynamic is often observed in dysfunctional family systems and can have long-lasting effects on the child's mental, emotional, and spiritual development (Chase 1999).[12]

A typical situation can be seen when the family consists of a single parent who struggles with chronic alcoholism and a 12-year-old child. Due to the parent's incapacity, the child takes on adult responsibilities. These include household chores, managing finances, and taking care of the parent during episodes of intoxication. The child also becomes the emotional caretaker, providing support and reassurance to the parent. They often comfort the parent, offer advice, or mediate conflicts. The child misses out on typical childhood experiences and may develop resentment, anxiety, and an exaggerated sense of responsibility. Their academic performance and social life may suffer as they prioritize family responsibilities over personal development.

Unfortunately, it is not uncommon to see *neglect and abuse* in a significantly dysfunctional family setting. This encompasses physical, emotional, or sexual abuse, as well as physical or emotional neglect. Abuse and neglect have profound and long-lasting effects on a person's psychological and emotional well-being (Herman 1997).[13]

Clinical Pastoral Counseling offers a faith-based approach to understanding and remedying family issues. Understanding these dynamics is crucial for counseling and therapeutic interventions to improve family relationships and individual well-being. Counseling often focuses on establishing healthy communication, setting appropriate boundaries, and addressing unique issues stemming from these dynamics (Clinton 2009).[14]

---

[12] Chase, N. D. (Ed.). (1999). "Burdened Children: Theory, Research, and Treatment of Parentification". Sage Publications.

[13] Herman, J. L. (1997). "Trauma and Recovery: The Aftermath of Violence - From Domestic Abuse to Political Terror". Basic Books.

[14] Clinton, T., & Hawkins, R. (2009). The Quick-Reference Guide to Biblical Counseling. Baker Books.

It is not uncommon to see negative family dynamics leading to compulsive or addictive processes. The family system is added to, whether in partnership or marriage, with the birth or addition of new family members. The system grows more extensive and more complex. With prolonged interactions come a network of beliefs, emotions, and behaviors.

The more positive the network or system, the more healthy and mature the cycle of beliefs, emotions, and behaviors. The more negative the family interactions, the more negatively impacted the family members' personalities, habits, perspectives, and interpretations.

While some in the family will comply, others rebel and escape. However, all become negatively affected and turn to run mechanisms to calm the angst. The healthier will turn to beneficial flights such as God, studying, work, activities, etc. The increasingly damaged character requires more instantly gratifying, dependable escapes to addictive behaviors.

Like a Cancer cell, the dysfunctional family begins with one self-protective and selfish person infecting the others within the family system. The infection often comes from fear and apprehension-based parent who exerts power and control to soothe themselves.

Other times, a significantly disturbed child learns to take control of the family by seeking negative attention, which in their troubled mind is better than no attention. The child or youth then infects the family system with fear and apprehension, leading others to anger and the need to protect both self and the rest of the family — retaliation.

Despite the cause, we activate the brain's basement of fear and apprehension (Limbic System). We are then turning off a higher level of good thinking skills in the brain's upper room (top half) — Dorsal Lateral Prefrontal Cortex DPLC.

From this point, our behavior is emotion-driven and impulsive. We have chosen not to reason through the problem. Instead, we are choosing to escape to the quick fix of self-protection and selfishness, which often leads us to some form of addictive behavior. The habit of the feel-good escape turns into a forceful urge (compulsion), which, if possible, leads to addiction.

Six Reasons Why Negative Family System Members Are More Susceptible To Addictive Behavior:

- They don't know how to have healthy relationships; "I don't need people."
- They haven't learned to trust; "No one is safe."
- They learn to distance themselves from people; "My addiction (needs) is more important than people or relationships."
- They are full of deep, lonely emptiness; "Life is meaningless; why bother."
- They know to treat people as objects; "My needs are more important."
- They default to the faulty belief system of a harmful lifestyle; "I can have whatever I want, whenever I want, no matter who I hurt."

The reinforcement of damage from dysfunctional family dynamics develops negative personality and behavioral changes. The resulting faulty beliefs lead to fixed delusions adapted through addictive escaping behavior.

The Bible Says...

". . . *A person actually reaps what they sow; a person actually receives the results of their own* **choices**. *The one who indulges the* **selfish nature** *will experience the* **natural consequences of a damaged mind** *— increased fear, broken relationships, separation from God, and eventual death [eternal separation from God]; but* **the one who chooses to follow the Spirit, from the Spirit they will experience a healed mind, internal peace, unity with God, and eternal life. So let us never become tired of living in harmony with God's methods of goodness,** *for if we don't turn back to self-destructive behaviors, we will—in time—experience a bountiful harvest. Therefore,* **at every opportunity, do good;** *and especially do good to other Christians so that God's principles may shine brightly in the church.*"
(Galatians 6:7-10 REM) (emphasis mine)

CHAPTER 3

ADULT CHILDREN OF
DYSFUNCTIONAL FAMILIES

There is a strong correlation between the adult children of addictive families and children of dysfunctional families. Many of the characteristics listed below are from the book *Adult Children of Alcoholics*.[15] I have adapted and added elements that give us a complete picture of the dysfunctional features often seen in people who come from disturbed families.

For the most part, there is no characteristic written in stone. When somebody chooses to improve themselves, healthier features will replace unhealthy ones. Many people develop addictive behavior because, in their dysfunctional family of origin, they learn to generate defensive and negative traits (fear & apprehension).

Adult Children of Dysfunctional Families ACODF is trying to heal their damaged minds, decrease fears, and build relationships. It is important to note that all individuals and families are somewhat dysfunctional, to a lesser or greater degree.

The Bible tells us that we are born with a sinful nature — a terminal illness — that often causes us to make decisions that are not good. To increase the right choices is to decrease the power of the sinful nature within us — the flesh.

---

[15] Woititz, Janet Geringer, (1983) "Adult Children of Alcoholics" Health Communications Inc.

"Therefore, the infection of distrust of God — which deformed humanity's heart and mind with selfishness and fear, and which results only in death — infected the human race when Adam accepted Satan's lies about God and broke trust with him. This infection of fear and selfishness is inherited by all human beings, so all are born infected." (Romans 5:12 REM)

God created spiritual rules or laws to organize our lives, just as God's Laws govern the universe (e.g., Law of Thermal Dynamics). God's spiritual laws are unchanging, unlike the routinely changing human laws. God gives us the freedom to follow His statutes and thrive or not.[16]

"For God so loved the world that He gave His only begotten Son, that whoever believes in Him should not perish but have everlasting life. For God did not send His Son into the world to condemn the people of the world, but that the people through Jesus can be saved…"

"…He who believes in Him is not condemned; but he who does not believe is condemned already, because he has not believed in the name of the only begotten Son of God. And this is the condemnation, that the light has come into the world, and men loved darkness rather than light, because their deeds were evil. For everyone practicing evil hates the light and does not come to the light, lest his deeds should be exposed. But he who does the truth comes to the light, that his deeds may be clearly seen, that they have been done in God." (John 3:16-21 NKJV)

The first step to change is admitting that something needs changing -- you will know if it needs replacing because it doesn't work. *"Your hearts must be cleansed and characters renewed, so that your lives bring forth actions in harmony with God's character of love."* (Matthew 3:8 REM)

If you are unhappy and relationships are not working for you, stop making the same mistakes repeatedly. It's time for a change! You may not have the power to change someone else, but our Creator has given you free will; you can improve yourself. The first step is a choice to change and seek help if needed.

"You were taught that the former ways of life—the survival-of-the-fittest

---

[16] Jennings, T., "The God Shaped Heart"

ways, the selfish me-first ways only lead to self-destruction and death, and that health and life consist of putting off such motives and desires. You were taught the importance of being recreated in heart and mind and displacing the principles of selfishness with those of love, and experiencing a complete transformation of character such that you are an entirely new being recreated in heart-attitude to be like God—truly righteous and holy." (Ephesians 4:22-24 REM)

Addictive Behavior Signs & Symptoms

People who display signs and symptoms of addictive behavior to a substance or behavior cannot control their use. They continue with compulsive behavior, even though it may cause harm (the individual may or may not be aware of the potential damage).

A sign refers to something others objectively observe or measure, representing facts. For example, signs of addictive behavior may be observing someone's compulsive (uncontrollable) gambling behavior or trembling hands. On the other hand, symptoms refer to feelings and concerns that can be perceived only by the person experiencing symptoms, such as subjective, intrusive (annoying) thoughts and feelings of the need to gamble.

The actor in addictive behavior can have powerful cravings but find it extremely difficult to stop without help.

The signs and symptoms of addictive behavior vary according to the individual, what they are addicted to, their family history (genetics), and personal circumstances.

The actor cannot stop; there will be at least one unsuccessful severe attempt to stop the addictive behavior.

The following are common signs & symptoms of addictive behavior:

- **Signs** and **symptoms** of withdrawal will occur where physical and mood-related discomfort becomes unbearable; frequently observed behaviors are severe moodiness, short temper, poor concentration, depression, emptiness, agitation, and bitterness.

- A sudden increase or decrease in appetite is characteristic of Addictive behavior.
- Insomnia or hypersomnia can occur.
- During addictive behavior, a person may experience severe constipation or diarrhea.
- Dynamic behavior can be exhibited by violence, trembling, seizures, hallucinations, and sweats.
- Addictive behavior will lead to declining health problems.
- Social or recreational sacrifices occur with addictive behavior taking priority.
- Addictive behavior will sacrifice genuine needs to maintain quick and easy access to their addiction.
- A higher level of risk-taking in addictive behavior.
- Addictive behavior requires the need for the addiction to deal with problems.
- When obsessing thoughts to access and protect the addiction.
- Increased lying, secrecy, and isolation are traits of addictive behavior.
- The actor will experience denial or delusional thoughts during addictive behavior — disturbed thinking.
- Addictive behavior will display excess use or abuse of the addiction use.
- Initial high use or intake to achieve a quick feel-good.
- Addictive behavior will lead to impaired judgment and legal problems.
- Financial difficulties accompany addictive behavior.
- Addictive behavior will result in severe relationship problems.

The Bible Says...

"My dear friends, since you are now part of God's kingdom, you are his ambassadors and representatives; therefore do not choose to indulge selfish and sinful desires, as such indulgence damages the mind and warps the character."
(1 Peter 2:11 REM)

CHAPTER 4

UNMASKING THE ADDICTIVE PERSONALITY

In exposing the true character of the stereotypical addict's personality, it is essential to understand three areas. *First,* addiction is a progressive illness that, left untreated, will increase in severity, damaging the body and brain. *Second,* addiction is a distorted relationship with an object or event. The concept of relationship is an intricate part of someone immersed in addiction. *Third,* the addictive process alters the personality. No matter how well-developed a person's personality, addiction will adversely change it. In this chapter, I describe an "active" addictive personality as someone currently engaged in substance or behavioral addiction.

The active, addictive personality can quickly become gravely passionate or attached to something or someone.

In and of itself, having an addictive personality is not bad. Having an addictive personality means being more alert to potentially harmful thoughts, feelings, and behaviors. Having an addictive personality does not mean someone will become an addict. The addictive personality indicates an inclination toward excess if boundaries are not established and adhered to.

In this series, we have given several definitions of addiction. Another description espoused by Craig Nakken (1996) is "Addiction

Is a pathological love and trust relationship with an object and/or event."[17]

The term pathological means abnormal compared to what is considered normal from the originating source of measurement. For example, as a Christian, my emotional and attachment needs come from God, who usually meets those needs through others. Meeting those needs is also accomplished through experiencing His Spirit's comforting inner peace. The Christian, caught up in the addictive cycle, tries to get those emotional and intimacy needs met, not through God but through objects and events.

The object can be a person because the active addictive personality does not view an individual as having unique needs. Instead, a "thing" (object) meets the addict's needs.

Several characteristics can help identify someone as having an active addictive personality, including:

- Binge eating or not eating to the point of harming the body
- Abuse or dependency of substances to cope, socialize, or relax
- Chronically checking one's cellphone or social media
- Frequent sexual encounters for a false sense of intimacy
- Compulsive buying or excessive shopping
- Gambling dependency or abuse
- Obsessing to the point of filling the mind to a troubling extent
- Excessive risk-taking
- Never feeling satisfied/needing more particular thoughts, feelings, or behaviors — Very quickly bored, demanding the FIX of CHANGE.
- An inability to curtail other harmful activities

An addictive personality developing abnormal (pathological) personality traits will exhibit maladaptive personality variants (fractured, disturbed, or distorted).

[17] Nakkan, Craig. (1996) The Addictive Personality, Hazelden Publications, Center City, Minnesota.

Five Negative Personality Dimensions of Addiction

The five negative personality dimensions are often evident when the active addictive personality becomes visible. Getting along with someone in active addiction can be very difficult and distressing. The absence of good features characterizes these five personality dimensions: negative emotions, detachment, antagonism, disinhibition (lack of restraint), and delusions (psychoticism).

Having a *Negative Emotion* is not seclusive to the addictive personality. Everyone will experience a few negative emotions during the day. The addictive personality in active addiction will occupy most of the day, discharging with negative emotions such as abandonment, shame, fear, powerlessness, invalidation, hopelessness, confusion, and bitterness. The pain of negative emotions can entice people to find themselves on a "self-medicating" path to addiction when using substances or behaviors to cope with painful feelings.

Detachment can be considered a physical experience of breaking contact with someone or something. Emotional detachment is the disconnect from others' emotions. In the active cycle of addiction, the addictive personality usually first detaches emotionally. The distancing of detachment is due to fear and apprehension of exposure or loss of their delusional love object or event — Rejecting before being rejected. Added stress increases the range of separation during detachment.

Antagonism in the active addictive personality is comparable to night and day; one moment, they are agreeable and friendly, and the next, they spout disagreeableness and bitterness. Narcissism, antisocially, impulsivity, manipulation, exploitation, and callousness are some defining traits of antagonism. Disagreeing with someone through negatively resisting is a far cry from respectfully disagreeing.

Disinhibition is unruly (unrestrained) behavior (frontal lobe slowing down) that results from lessening or losing the fear of consequences and disregarding spiritual/cultural/social constraints.

For example, we may tell our children not to curse. However, after hearing others cursing throughout the day (and from their TV programs), the children can become disinhibited and begin "cursing like a sailor" because of the **fear of rejection** if seen as different.

Unrestrained behavior (disinhibition) and significant impulsiveness are loss of standard control in the brain's complex thinking region (Frontal Lobe). For the active addictive personality, there is a powering down of electrical and blood flow, hindering the frontal lobe from problem-solving.

Unlike disinhibition, the fear of painful consequences will cause many to "inhibit" behaviors (either consciously or unconsciously).

Delusions can be a mild form of psychosis, believing a lie to be true despite a weight of evidence to the contrary — Impairment of interpreting or reasoning (Denial). Delusions are persistent and intrusive false beliefs not swayed by reason or senses. (see Jeremiah 10:15, 51:18; James 1:22; 1 Thessalonians 2:3; 2 Thessalonians 2:11)

The Bible speaks of delusions as lies misperceived and rigidly accepted as truths.

The Bible Says...

"I am frustrated with what I do! For having been restored to trust, I want to do what is in harmony with God and his methods and principles; but I find that even though I trust God, my old habits, conditioned responses, preconceived ideas and other remnants of the devastation caused by distrust and selfishness are not yet fully removed. And if I find an old habit causing me to behave in ways that I now find detestable, I affirm that the law is a very helpful tool revealing residual damage in need of healing. What is happening is this: I have come to trust God, and I desire to do his will, but old habits and conditioned responses — which present almost reflexively in certain situations — have not yet been totally eliminated and thus cause me to do things I do not want to do."

(Romans 7:15-17 REM)

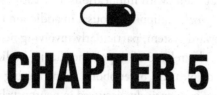

CHAPTER 5

THREE LEVELS OF INTOXICATION

Three Types of Highs in the Active Addictive Personality

As stated earlier, having an addictive personality does not mean someone will become an addict. If a substance or behavioral disorder occurs, I have identified the addictive personality as being in an active stage of addiction. An active addictive personality is in a "disease" state affecting the brain and behavior. The disease leads to an inability to fully control oneself despite the harm done by substances or behaviors.

During substance and behavioral addictions, the addictive personality moves into three types of elevated experiences: arousal, satiation, and fantasy.

Arousal

The arousal state in addictive personalities is a complex interplay of biological, psychological, behavioral, and social factors. Understanding these components is essential for developing comprehensive approaches to treatment and prevention.

The "arousal" state in the context of addictive personalities refers to a heightened physiological and psychological condition that is often associated with anticipation or engagement in addictive behaviors. This state can be understood through various psychological theories and research findings involving biological, psychological, behavioral, social & environmental, along with implications for treatment.

From a *biological* standpoint, arousal in addiction is closely linked to the brain's reward system, particularly involving neurotransmitters like dopamine. The release of dopamine during addictive behaviors creates a sense of pleasure or euphoria, contributing to the arousal state. This process is extensively discussed in neuropsychology (Volkow 2016).[18]

From the *psychological* perspective (mental and emotional), arousal in addiction is often linked to the concept of "cue-induced" cravings. This is where environmental or emotional cues trigger intense arousal states, leading to cravings and potentially addictive behavior (Witkiewitz 2013).[19]

Behaviorally, the arousal state in addiction can also be understood through classical and operant conditioning models. Addictive substances or behaviors are often initially engaged in due to their pleasurable effects (positive reinforcement) or their ability to alleviate negative states (negative reinforcement), leading to heightened arousal states when anticipating these outcomes (Hyman 2005).[20]

Social and environmental factors also play a significant role in the arousal state of addictive personalities. The social context can influence arousal states by facilitating or inhibiting addictive behaviors (Kelly 2010).[21]

---

[18] Volkow, N. D., Koob, G. F., & McLellan, A. T. (2016). Neurobiologic Advances from the Brain Disease Model of Addiction. New England Journal of Medicine, 374(4), 363–371. https://doi.org/10.1056/NEJMra1511480.

[19] Witkiewitz, K., Lustyk, M. K. B., & Bowen, S. (2013). Retraining the Addicted Brain: A Review of Hypothesized Neurobiological Mechanisms of Mindfulness-Based Relapse Prevention. Psychology of Addictive Behaviors, 27(2), 351–365. https://doi.org/10.1037/a0029258.

[20] Hyman, S. E. (2005). Addiction: A Disease of Learning and Memory. American Journal of Psychiatry, 162(8), 1414–1422. https://doi.org/10.1176/appi.ajp.162.8.1414.

[21] Kelly, J. F., & Westerhoff, C. M. (2010). Does it matter how we refer to individuals with substance-related conditions? A randomized study of two commonly used terms. International Journal of Drug Policy, 21(3), 202–207. https://doi.org/10.1016/j.drugpo.2009.10.010.

Grasping the implications of treatment is essential for developing effective treatment strategies. For instance, cognitive-behavioral therapy (CBT) often targets the cognitive processes associated with arousal and cravings. Mindfulness-based interventions also aim to regulate arousal states by increasing awareness and control over reactions to cravings (Garland 2014).[22]

Arousal is a feeling of strength and authority, which uplifts an individual's confidence, self-promotion, and exploitation. This sensation of arousal leads those susceptible to addiction to believe that they can attain security, satisfaction, and significance by gaining control over their circumstances.

However, while experiencing this empowerment, they unknowingly deplete their true power. As inevitable fear and apprehension begin to accumulate, individuals with active addictive personalities seek even more power through additional arousal.

As the active addictive personality becomes increasingly aware of the need for more substances or behaviors to maintain their sense of power, their fear of being exposed as powerless intensifies.

To restore their sense of arousal, individuals with active addictive personalities turn to familiar substances or behaviors. Such substances may include amphetamines, cocaine, ecstasy/speed, or alcohol. At the same time, arousal-seeking behaviors may involve engaging in sexual acts, gambling, compulsive spending, dishonesty, theft, seeking out stress, chaos, conflict, and more.

Satiation

Understanding "satiation" in the context of an addictive personality involves exploring how individuals with addictive tendencies perceive and react to the fulfillment of their desires or needs. In substance and behavioral addiction, satiation can be elusive, as the addictive behavior

---

[22] Garland, E. L., Froeliger, B., & Howard, M. O. (2014). Mindfulness training targets neurocognitive mechanisms of addiction at the attention-appraisal-emotion interface. Frontiers in Psychiatry, 4, 173. https://doi.org/10.3389/fpsyt.2013.00173.

often falls to provide lasting satisfaction, leading to a repetitive cycle of behavior seeking that elusive fulfillment.

Satiation in psychology refers to being fully satisfied or gratified to the extent that the desire or need for a particular stimulus is diminished or temporarily ceased. For someone with an addictive personality, achieving satiation is often challenging. The addiction typically involves a compulsive engagement in rewarding stimuli despite adverse consequences. This lack of satiation can be understood through the lens of **reward deficiency syndrome**, which suggests that individuals with certain genetic predispositions may have a blunted response to typical rewards, leading them to seek excessive stimulation or engagement in addictive behaviors (Blum et al., 2000).[23]

Dopamine, a neurotransmitter linked to the brain's reward system, plays a crucial role in addiction and the concept of satiation. In addictive personalities, the dopamine response to addictive substances or behaviors is often heightened initially. Still, over time, the individual may require more substance or behavior to achieve the same level of satisfaction, a phenomenon known as **tolerance** (Volkow et al., 2016).[24]

Psychological theories, such as the cognitive-behavioral model, suggest that addictive behaviors are partly driven by dysfunctional beliefs and thoughts that disrupt the natural satiation process. Individuals with addictive personalities may have cognitive distortions that lead them to overvalue the addictive behavior and undervalue the negative consequences (Beck et al., 1993).[25]

Treatment approaches for addictive personalities often focus on re-establishing a sense of satiation through healthier means. Cognitive-behavioral therapy (CBT) and mindfulness-based interventions are

[23] Blum, K., Braverman, E. R., Holder, J. M., Lubar, J. F., Monastra, V. J., Miller, D., ... & Comings, D. E. (2000). Reward deficiency syndrome: a biogenetic model for the diagnosis and treatment of impulsive, addictive, and compulsive behaviors. Journal of Psychoactive Drugs, 32(supl), 1-112.

[24] Volkow, N. D., Koob, G. F., & McLellan, A. T. (2016). Neurobiologic Advances from the Brain Disease Model of Addiction. New England Journal of Medicine, 374(4), 363-371.

[25] Beck, A. T., Wright, F. D., Newman, C. F., & Liese, B. S. (1993). Cognitive therapy of substance abuse. Guilford press.

commonly used to help individuals recognize and modify the thought patterns that contribute to the addictive cycle, aiming to restore a more balanced and realistic assessment of what brings satisfaction (Witkiewitz et al., 2005).[26]

Satiation in the context of addictive personalities is often unachievable through the addictive behavior alone. It involves biological, psychological, and social factors that interact in ways that perpetuate the addiction cycle. Understanding and addressing these factors is critical to effective treatment and recovery.

Satiation is characterized by achieving a state of overindulgence or fulfillment of a specific need. The diminishing effectiveness of a reinforcer marks this phenomenon due to its frequent exposure (Koob 2016).[27] Such satiation often culminates in a growing dissatisfaction towards a person, place, or thing, epitomized by sentiments like "I don't feel anything for you anymore."

This process triggers a mental, emotional, and physiological response where the mind and body strive to reestablish a sense of normalcy, often through a rebound effect. This rebounding manifests as an addictive ritual, which paradoxically leads to increased pain and dissatisfaction, essentially creating a situation with no positive outcome (Doweiko 2015).[28]

Interestingly, the grieving process associated with this cycle can begin even before reaching satiation. The anticipation of returning dissatisfaction can give rise to a plethora of emotional and psychological challenges, including anxiety, panic, confusion, feelings of invalidation, bitterness, despair (often manifesting as depression), and self-destructive behaviors (Goodman 1993).[29]

To attain satiation, individuals with an addictive personality

---

[26] Witkiewitz, K., Marlatt, G. A., & Walker, D. (2005). Mindfulness-based relapse prevention for alcohol and substance use disorders. Journal of Cognitive Psychotherapy, 19(3), 211-228.

[27] Koob, G. F., & Volkow, N. D. (2016). Neurobiology of addiction: A neurocircuitry analysis. *Lancet Psychiatry, 3*(8), 760-773. doi:10.1016/S2215-0366(16)00104-8

[28] Doweiko, H. E. (2015). Concepts of chemical dependency. Cengage Learning.

[29] Goodman, A. (1993). Diagnosis and treatment of sexual addiction. *Journal of Sex & Marital Therapy, 19*(3), 225-251. doi:10.1080/00926239308404908

frequently turn to familiar substances or behaviors. Common substances include various opiates such as Opium, Codeine, Morphine, Darvon, Heroin, and Methadone, among others, as well as alcohol. On the behavioral front, typical methods for seeking satiation include overeating, alcohol intoxication, and engaging in excessive exercise (which releases endorphins), thereby inducing an artificial sense of well-being and numbing emotional or physical pain.

"Because Opioid withdrawal symptoms can seem so frightening to users, fear can keep them from using. For many long-term users, the fear of withdrawal becomes a greater trigger for continued use than the desire to repeat the 'rush.'"[30]

Fantasy

Understanding the role of "fantasy" in the context of addictive personalities involves delving into the psychological mechanisms that drive addictive behaviors. The concept of fantasy, in this context, refers to the mental and emotional escapism that individuals with addictive personalities often seek, which can reinforce or exacerbate their addictive behaviors.

Fantasy serves as a form of *escapism* for many individuals with addictive personalities. This escapism is about avoiding real-life challenges and seeking pleasure or relief in an imagined world that feels more controllable and satisfying than reality. For example, a study by Sussman et al. (2011) highlighted that individuals with addictive personalities often engage in activities that offer escape, including substance abuse, gambling, or excessive internet use.[31]

Fantasizing can activate the brain's reward pathways, similar to the effects of addictive substances. *Dopamine*, a neurotransmitter associated with pleasure and reward, is often released during fantasy-based

---

[30] Inaba, Darryl, et.al., Uppers, Downers, All Arounders, Third Edition, p. 147, CNS Publications Inc., Ashland, OR, 1997.

[31] Sussman, S., Lisha, N., & Griffiths, M. (2011). Prevalence of the Addictions: A Problem of the Majority or the Minority? *Evaluation & the Health Professions, 34*(1), 3-56. doi:10.1177/0163278710380124

activities, reinforcing the behavior. Kühn and Gallinat (2014), in their study on the impact of internet pornography on the brain, noted that the fantasy elements in such material could stimulate dopamine production, mirroring addiction patterns.[32]

Highly fantasy-prone individuals might be more susceptible to addictive behaviors. A *fantasy-prone personality* is one where a person has a vivid and deep engagement with their inner imaginative world. This disposition can increase the likelihood of substance abuse and other addictive behaviors as a means of augmenting or escaping into their fantasy world. Merckelbach et al. (2001) discussed how high levels of fantasy proneness are related to dissociative tendencies, which can be linked to addictive behaviors.[33]

Curiously, fantasy can also be harnessed in therapeutic settings to help individuals with addictive personalities. Techniques such as guided imagery and visualization can be used in therapy to help patients overcome addictive impulses by redirecting their focus to more positive and constructive fantasies. This approach is highlighted in the work of Singer and Singer (2006), who discussed the therapeutic use of daydreaming and imagination in coping with addictions.[34]

The role of fantasy in addictive personality serves both as a pathway to addictive behaviors and as a potential tool for *therapeutic intervention*. The ability of imagination to provide an escape from reality while stimulating the brain's reward systems makes it a significant factor in understanding and treating addictive personalities. However, when guided and controlled, the exact mechanism can also be utilized positively in counseling settings to aid recovery and rehabilitation.

In therapeutic settings, particularly in Christian counseling contexts, it is beneficial to explore how spiritual practices and faith-based

---

[32] Kühn, S., & Gallinat, J. (2014). Brain Structure and Functional Connectivity Associated With Pornography Consumption: The Brain on Porn. *JAMA Psychiatry, 71*(7), 827-834. doi:10.1001/jamapsychiatry.2014.93

[33] Merckelbach, H., Horselenberg, R., & Muris, P. (2001). The Creative Experiences Questionnaire (CEQ): a brief self-report measure of fantasy proneness. *Personality and Individual Differences, 31*(6), 987-995. doi:10.1016/s0191-8869(00)00201-4

[34] Singer, J. L., & Singer, D. G. (2006). Imagination and Play in the Electronic Age. Harvard University Press.

perspectives can aid in addressing the root causes of fantasy as a form of escapism in addictive personalities. Integrating spiritual guidance with mental and emotional interventions can offer a holistic approach to healing and recovery.

When in a state of Fantasy, the active addictive personality will experience confusion and a sense of depersonalization; "An altered sense of the reality of one's surroundings or oneself (e.g., seeing oneself from another's perspective, being in a daze, time slowing)."[35]

In Fantasy, the active addictive personality uses typical substances or behaviors. Some examples of substances are Psychedelics such as LSD, Mushrooms, Peyote, Belladonna, PCP, & Marijuana. The example behaviors used for fantasy are daydreaming and rituals, which lead to a trance-like state of mind — a half-conscious state between sleeping and waking. —Timothy Leary said, "To use your head, you have to go out of your mind!"[36]

A trancelike state of mind can be as simple as repetitive daily activities requiring movements with little awareness. However, to the actively addictive personality, semiconsciousness can make them unaware (not clear) of their thoughts, attitudes, and behaviors, and speaking those famous last words, "I don't remember that." Or, they are often just lying, and it's hard for a loving partner to tell the difference!

The Bible Says...

"Since we suffer with the same sickness of heart and mind as they did [by grumbling and complaining], all of this history is recorded for our benefit—to warn and protect us—so we won't refuse as they did, but will fulfill God's purpose of victorious living at this present time. So, if you are in God's treatment program and believe you are doing well, be careful that you don't fall behind in your appointments with God, or in the partaking

[35] Diagnostic and Statistical Manual of Mental Disorders, Fifth Edition, Text Revision (DSM-5-TR), p. 314, American Psychiatric Association, Washington, D.C., 2022

[36] Retrieved from https://quotefancy.com/quote/1002516/Timothy-Leary-To-use-your-head-you-have-to-go-out-of-your-mind.

of his Remedy. For there is no temptation to discontinue God's treatment that has come upon you except for the fear and selfishness that infects all mankind. God is reliable and trustworthy; he will not allow temptation beyond your ability to resist, but when you are tempted, he will always provide resources, options, opportunities, supports, and alternate ways out so that you can stand your ground and overcome the temptation, thereby growing stronger with each victory…We demolish every idea, argument, doctrine, teaching or concept that infects the mind and distorts or obstructs the truth about God, and we reclaim the thoughts, feelings and attitudes into the truth about God as revealed by Jesus Christ."

(1 Corinthians 10:11-13, 10:5 REM) (brackets added; pjs)

CHAPTER 6

THE ADDICTIVE PERSONALITY AND RELATIONSHIPS

Can The "Active" Addictive Personality Have Genuine Human-To-Human Relationships?

Explaining the impediments to a loving human-to-human relationship when one or both persons have an addictive personality can be challenging. Since God designed each of us with unique characteristics, addiction introduces complexity and difficulty in achieving relational satisfaction. We can examine how addiction impacts interpersonal dynamics. Addiction, whether to substances or behaviors, often leads to a range of mental, emotional, and behavioral changes that can significantly strain relationships. Let's examine eight of the multiple issues arising in addictive personality relationships.

Trust issues are usually the first to come up in marital counseling. Addiction can lead to dishonesty and secretive behavior as the addicted individual might lie about their addiction or actions related to it. This trust erosion undermines any relationship's foundation, making open and honest communication difficult (Rotunda et al., 2004).[37]

Individuals struggling with addiction may become *emotionally*

---

[37] Rotunda, R. J., West, L., & O'Farrell, T. J. (2004). Enabling behavior in a clinical sample of alcohol-dependent clients and their partners. Journal of Substance Abuse Treatment, 26(4), 269-276.

unavailable or neglectful of their partner's and family's needs. The preoccupation with the addictive substance or behavior can lead to neglecting emotional connections and responsibilities within the relationship (McCrady & Epstein, 2009).[38]

Relationships involving addiction often become *codependent,* with the non-addicted partner enabling the addictive behavior, either knowingly or unknowingly. This dynamic can create a cycle that is hard to break and can be damaging to both individuals (Cermak, T. M., 1986).[39]

Addiction can lead to increased *conflict,* aggression, and, in some cases, *abuse.* Substance abuse, in particular, is associated with a higher risk of domestic violence (O'Farrell & Fals-Stewart, 2006).[40]

Addictions can be expensive to maintain, leading to *financial* difficulties, which are a common source of stress and conflict in relationships (Morgenstern et al., 2001).[41]

The *health problems* associated with addiction, whether physical or mental, can place a significant burden on the relationship. The partner may become more of a caregiver than a romantic partner, leading to resentment and burnout (Orford et al., 2005).[42]

Addiction will severely impact sexual and emotional *intimacy.* Issues such as decreased sexual desire, performance issues, or infidelity

---

[38] McCrady, B. S., & Epstein, E. E. (2009). Overcoming alcohol problems: A couples-focused program. Oxford University Press.

[39] Cermak, T. M. (1986). Diagnosing and treating co-dependence: A guide for professionals who work with chemical dependents, their spouses, and children. Johnson Institute Books.

[40] O'Farrell, T. J., & Fals-Stewart, W. (2006). Behavioral couples therapy for alcoholism and drug abuse. Guilford Press.

[41] Morgenstern, J., Blanchard, K. A., Morgan, T. J., Labouvie, E., & Hayaki, J. (2001). Testing the effectiveness of cognitive-behavioral treatment for substance abuse in a community setting: Within treatment and posttreatment findings. Journal of Consulting and Clinical Psychology, 69(6), 1007-1017.

[42] Orford, J., Natera, G., Copello, A., Atkinson, C., Mora, J., Velleman, R., ... & Tiburcio, M. (2005). Coping with alcohol and drug problems: The experiences of family members in three contrasting cultures. Routledge.

related to addictive behaviors can arise, further complicating the relationship (Schneider & Irons 2001).[43]

In counseling, addressing these issues requires a nuanced understanding of the interplay between addiction and relationship dynamics.

Interventions often involve not just the treatment of the addiction itself but also couples therapy to address the relational issues that have arisen as a result (O'Farrell & Clements 2012).[44]

The Love Triangle of Science, Scripture, and Experience

The essence of human relationships can be visualized as a triangle with three essential corners: Science, Scripture, and Experience. Love flourishes when relationships are built upon these three pillars of divine truth. However, when love falters, it is often because one or more of these foundational supports are not evidenced.

Before delving into the support corners of the relational triangle, let's remind ourselves that all of us are born with a selfish, carnal nature — sin (Psalm 51:5; Romans 3:23, 5:12; Genesis 6:5). We did not choose to be born in selfishness. *"Surely I was sinful at birth, sinful from the time my mother conceived me."* (Psalms 51:5 NIV) Healthy relationships cannot thrive in an environment of selfishness. The question is, "What will we do about it?"

"Those who live with the selfish nature in charge have their minds bent on self-indulgence and selfish pursuits; but those who live in harmony with the Spirit of truth and love have their minds focused on living in harmony with God's principles of truth, love, and liberty. The mind of the selfish person is filled with death, but the mind governed by the principles of the Spirit of truth and love is filled with life and peace. The selfish mind operates on the survival-of-the-fittest principle, which says, 'I love myself so

---

[43] Schneider, J. P., & Irons, R. R. (2001). Sex, lies, and forgiveness: Couples speaking out on healing from sex addiction. Hazelden.

[44] O'Farrell, T. J., & Clements, K. (2012). Review of outcome research on marital and family therapy in treatment for alcoholism. Journal of Marital and Family Therapy, 38(1), 122-144.

much that I will kill you in order that I may live;' and such a mind is at war with the God of love, who says, 'I love you so much that I will give my life in order that you might live.' The mind of the selfish person does not surrender to the principle of love—which requires death to self-interest—nor can it do so; those controlled by the selfish nature cannot please God, because everything they do is opposed to all that God is." (Romans 8:5-8 REM)

The active addictive personality (AAP) takes selfishness to an extreme because it is a condition of the heart and mind that is out of harmony with God and His kingdom of love. The state of addiction fractures love and trust, resulting in fear, apprehension, self-protection, and selfishness. There is no room for meeting others' intimacy needs, e.g., acceptance or respect, to secure a healthy bond.[45]

Science, The First Triangle Support Corner

Believe it or not, a relationship's first triangle support corner is *Science*. The Scientific method is a body of techniques for investigating phenomena based on verifiable or measurable evidence subject to logic and reasoning principles.

God's law of Love can be seen through the lens of Science as the principle of giving upon which all life is built. As we inhale oxygen produced by other living organisms (e.g., plants) —Law of Respiration—we exhale carbon dioxide (CO_2) to other organisms, such as plants, that reciprocate the cycle. However, if you break the cycle by covering your head in plastic wrap and stop breathing, the plants will die, and the earth will grow cold without greenhouse gas (CO_2).

Each time the AAP participates in their addiction, damage occurs in neuron clusters. Intelligence decreases while poor impulse control and selfishness increase.

When giving ceases, life stops. Living organisms are interdependent, requiring simultaneous giving — God's Design Law of Love. God's Law of Love and other Laws (e.g., Laws of Respiration, Exertion, Gravity...,

---

[45] Request Dr. Samaan's list of thirty intimacy needs: healing@ newhorizonscounseling.org

etc.) are measurable and confirm Science proves that order requires the process of intelligence. The relational triangle supports the corner of Science evidence matter, energy, and coded information (DNA). *"…be united in love, purpose, motive, method, and constant care and concern for each other. Don't do anything for selfish reasons or seek to promote yourself ahead of others, but in humbleness and love, be more concerned for the welfare and good of others than for your own. Each one of you should not only be concerned with your health and growth but also work to help others become the healthiest Christians they can be."* (Philippians 2:3b-4 REM)

The Bible Says…

"When the selfish nature is in charge, it is obvious, because the life reflects the destructive behaviors of the selfish nature,…All such behaviors destroy the image of God in humankind, dethrone reason, sear the conscience, inflame the debasing desires, and result in individuals—although created in God's image—digressing into nonthinking, animalistic brutes incapable of entering the kingdom of God." (Galatians 5:19-21 REM)

"But when the time was right, God intervened and sent his Son—born of a sin-infected human mother, as a real human baby, with a humanity weakened by the law of sin and death — in order to purify, cleanse and purge humanity from the infection of selfishness and fear. He did this in order to heal and restore those diagnosed as "terminal" by the written law, so that we might receive all the blessings of sons and daughters of God. Because we are children of God, God sent the Spirit of his Son into our hearts to restore Christlikeness of character so that we genuinely call out to God, "Daddy, Father!" Rejoice! You are no longer childlike, needing the supervision of a slave, but are adult children, wise and mature; and as mature children—heirs with Christ of all that is promised!" (Galatians 4:4-7 REM)

The Support Corner of Scripture

Scripture can be seen as another relational support corner of the triangle revealing God's love character. Our Creator God did not selfishly hold on to power but surrendered power, position, and prestige to become our Savior in the man Jesus Christ. Jesus accomplished His mission by revealing God to the followers (John 14:9, 17:6; 1 Peter 1:18). He suffered and died to reach us with HIS love, the opposite of an actively addictive personality (AAP). *"And after becoming human, he voluntarily humbled himself to perfectly reveal God's character of love, choosing to love at all costs. He wouldn't even use his power to prevent his death on the cross; thus, he overcame selfishness with love!"* (Philippians 2:8 REM)

The essence of God is consistently described as love, a notion that remains constant across all temporal dimensions—past, present, and future. This idea aligns with the scriptural assertion in 1 Corinthians 13, where love is selfless, a quality that never deviates. Just as love perpetually avoids self-seeking, so does God, embodying this attribute in all aspects of His existence.

As the Creator, God has infused the entirety of creation with this intrinsic nature of love. This is evident in how He brought the universe into existence and actively maintained it, continually offering a part of Himself in the process. This foundational principle of love underpins God's law, serving as a divine blueprint that governs the natural order. This law ensures the harmony and sustenance of all creation, reflecting God's unwavering commitment to love (Jennings 2011).[46]

The role of the Bible Scriptures in relationship building is crucial. Emphasizing love and compassion guides individuals toward nurturing and maintaining healthy relationships. This is articulated in the works of authors such as Townsend and Cloud (1995), who emphasize the importance of biblical principles in forming and sustaining interpersonal bonds.[47]

The concept that addictive personalities may bond with substances

---

[46] Jennings, T. (2011) "God is Love — All The Time." https://comeandreason.com/god-is-love-all-the-time/

[47] Townsend, J., & Cloud, H. (1995). Safe People: How to Find Relationships That Are Good for You and Avoid Those That Aren't. Zondervan.

ᴏɪ behaviors instead of people is discussed in-depth by scholars like Carnes (2001). He explores how the absence of nurturing relationships can lead individuals towards addictive behaviors as a form of coping mechanism.[48]

Love is a crucial element in relationships. Chapman (2015) explores the necessity of love for healthy relationship building, detailing how love is pivotal in forming and maintaining meaningful connections.[49]

Being so self-involved, the active addictive personality (AAP) will take from the needs of others to continue in their terminal addictive lifestyle. The AAP cannot comprehend sacrificial love, the power source that keeps the fires of passion burning.

Love exists in freedom (liberty). Demonstrating God's unconditional love, Jesus showed that He would rather die than selfishly use His power to take away our self-determination. *"For God loved the world so much that he gave me, his One and only Son, so that all who open their hearts and trust me will be healed, and therefore not perish but have everlasting life."* (John 3:16 REM)

The AAP loses meaning and hope through fear, invalidation, powerlessness, loss of identity and individuality, bitterness, and the failure of healthy thinking. Those who have persisted in their addictive lifestyle destroy their faculties sensitive to the movements of truth and love. AAPs settle themselves into lies, wrong behaviors, rebellion, and opposition.

The relational support corner of Scripture provides a truthful relationship with meaning and hope. Scripture teaches us to envision a better life, leading to immortal life. Jesus is giving the image of a world restored to sinless perfection, with no fear, selfishness, exploitation, sickness, pain, suffering, or death. The triangle relational support corner of Scripture shows us a world where everyone loves others more than themselves.

"So come to me, all who are tired, worn down and exhausted from

---

[48] Carnes, P. (2001). Out of the Shadows: Understanding Sexual Addiction. Hazelden Publishing.

[49] Chapman, G. (2015). The 5 Love Languages: The Secret to Love that Lasts. Northfield Publishing.

fear, selfishness, and fighting to survive on your own, and I will give you rest. Join up with me and learn my methods—the principles upon which life is built to operate—for I am gentle and humble in heart, and you will find healing and rest for your souls. For joining up with me and living in harmony with the way life is designed to operate is what makes life easy and lightens life's burdens." (Matthew 11:28-30 REM)

In contrast to the active addictive personality (AAP), which focuses on self-protection, genuine love is portrayed in the Bible as the unification of a disciple with Christ, much like a branch connected to a vine. Remaining in Christ guarantees bearing fruit, not merely as a possibility, but as a certainty. Jesus implores his followers to stay in his love, assuring them that he loves them just as the Father loves him. One way to abide in his love is through obedience to his commands, mirroring his obedience to the Father's commands. According to Jesus, adherence defines love rather than an emotional sentiment. The believer's joy doesn't stem from an easy life but from a life entirely devoted to Christ. To the AAP, this helps take the focus off the self, teaching love to the loveless.

Throughout his ministry, from the beginning until the resurrection, Jesus consistently taught his disciples the importance of loving one another. The benchmark for this love is Christ's love. He would ultimately demonstrate this love through his death, which is evident in his close friendship and trust with his disciples. Jesus chose and appointed them to be his messengers, fully aware that they would bear lasting fruit as they lived a life dedicated to his mission. In this context, bearing fruit is closely tied to evangelism and the fulfillment of answered prayers. Believers are encouraged to lay their hearts bare when they pray. Selfish or worldly desires should not drive their prayers but encompass all aspects of their lives. Their prayers are guided by God's Word and focus on bringing Christ glory.

"As the Father has loved me, so have I loved you. Now remain in my love. If you keep my commands, you will remain in my love, just as I have kept my Father's commands and remain in his love. I have told you this so that my joy may be in you and that your joy may be complete. My command is this: Love each other as I have loved you. Greater love has no

one than this: to lay down one's life for one's friends. You are my friends if you do what I command. I no longer call you servants, because a servant does not know his master's business. Instead, I have called you friends, for everything that I learned from my Father I have made known to you. You did not choose me, but I chose you and appointed you so that you might go and bear fruit—fruit that will last—and so that whatever you ask in my name the Father will give you. This is my command: Love each other." (John 15:9-17 NIV)

The triangular cornerstone of Scripture plays an indispensable role in fortifying human relationships. This biblical foundation is essential for nurturing interpersonal connections. In its absence, individuals with addictive tendencies struggle to develop healthy bonding abilities. Rather than forming bonds with people, they often gravitate towards inanimate objects, substances, and harmful behaviors. This maladaptive bonding can be attributed to a lack of love and emotional support, which is critical for healthy relationship development.

The Junction of Experience

The junction of "experience" in insight, particularly in the context of an addictive personality, involves an interplay of cognitive, emotional, and behavioral processes. Addiction often disrupts the normal learning process, which is where experience typically contributes to the development of wisdom. However, in individuals with addictive personalities, this learning process can be hindered, leading to repeated mistakes despite adverse consequences.

Cognitive Aspects

Active addictive personalities (AAP) often exhibit *cognitive distortions*, such as denial, rationalization, and minimization. These distortions can impair the individual's ability to gain insight from experiences. Insight in this context refers to the self-awareness and understanding necessary to recognize these distortions and learn from past mistakes (Beck et al., 1993).[50]

Addiction can affect *memory and learning* processes, which are essential for gaining insight from experiences. Substance abuse, for instance, can impair the brain's ability to encode, store, and retrieve memories, thus impacting the learning of lessons from past behaviors (Volkow et al., 2016).[51]

Emotional Aspects

Addictive personalities often struggle with *emotional dysregulation*, which can impede the process of learning from experiences. The intense emotional states associated with addiction can overshadow the cognitive processing of experiences, leading to repeated mistakes (Koob & Le Moal, 2008).[52]

Mindfulness-based interventions can enhance *emotional awareness*, allowing individuals to experience their emotions without judgment and develop insight. This process aids in breaking the cycle of addiction by fostering a deeper understanding of one's emotional triggers and responses (Witkiewitz et al., 2013).[53]

Behavioral Aspects

Addictive behaviors can become deeply ingrained *habits* driven more by *compulsion* than conscious choice. This habitual nature can make it

---

[50] Beck, A. T., Wright, F. D., Newman, C. F., & Liese, B. S. (1993). *Cognitive therapy of substance abuse.* Guilford Press.

[51] Volkow, N. D., Koob, G. F., & McLellan, A. T. (2016). Neurobiologic Advances from the Brain Disease Model of Addiction. *New England Journal of Medicine, 374,* 363–371.

[52] Koob, G. F., & Le Moal, M. (2008). Addiction and the brain antireward system. *Annual Review of Psychology, 59,* 29–53.

[53] Witkiewitz, K., Lustyk, M. K. B., & Bowen, S. (2013). Retraining the addicted brain: A review of hypothesized neurobiological mechanisms of mindfulness-based relapse prevention. *Psychology of Addictive Behaviors, 27*(2), 351–365.

challenging to apply insights gained from past experiences to current behavior (Everitt & Robbins 2005).[54]

Cognitive-behavioral therapy (CBT) and Transformation Prayer Ministry (TPM)[55] aim to modify maladaptive behaviors by integrating insights from past experiences into current decision-making processes. This approach can help individuals recognize patterns and consciously work to change them (McHugh, Hearon, & Otto, 2010).[56]

The journey toward wisdom requires a deep understanding of the interplay between experience and insight, especially for individuals with addictive personalities. By acknowledging the cognitive, emotional, and behavioral aspects at play, we can begin to untangle the complexities of our behaviors and make better choices moving forward. Let us not disrupt the natural process of learning and growth but instead embrace every opportunity to gain wisdom.

Through continued learning, we can transcend the adverse consequences of repeated mistakes and pave the path toward a more fulfilling and enlightened existence. As we embark on this journey, may we draw inspiration from the truth and guidance in the Bible, knowing that with God's grace, we can overcome any obstacle and find true wisdom. Commit yourselves to this noble pursuit, and may it lead to a life of purpose, fulfillment, and everlasting joy.

Spiritual and Holistic Considerations

The integration of spiritual insights can play a significant role in Christian counseling. Understanding and learning from experiences may also involve a spiritual dimension, where individuals seek guidance

---

[54] Everitt, B. J., & Robbins, T. W. (2005). Neural systems of reinforcement for drug addiction: From actions to habits to compulsion. *Nature Neuroscience, 8*(11), 1481–1489.

[55] Smith, E., Smith, J. (2018) "Effortless Forgiveness." New Creation Publishing, Campbellsville, KY.

[56] McHugh, R. K., Hearon, B. A., & Otto, M. W. (2010). Cognitive-Behavioral Therapy for Substance Use Disorders. *Psychiatric Clinics of North America, 33*(3), 511–525.

and wisdom through prayer, meditation, and scriptural study. This spiritual insight can provide additional strength and perspective in overcoming addictive behaviors and learning from past experiences (McMinn, 2011).[57]

Knowledge is a good thing, and understanding knowledge is even better. However, without the junction of experience, there can be no insight (Wisdom) to stop from repeating mistakes.

The out-of-control AAP requires human law to diagnose defects, treat them, and quarantine them, and it will require governance. The selfish nature will grow too powerful for self-governance and will require intervention.

Whether learning the experience through the events of others or a personal loss, we find that God's principles heal — His principles work. Experiencing God's healing comes through the outgrowth of love, joy, peace, patience, kindness, goodness, trustworthiness, gentleness, and self-control (Galatians 5:22-23 NIV). [a picture of complete self-governess]

While experiencing inpatient or outpatient treatment programs is beneficial, an eager and active participant is still required. God's principles heal when we trust Him, embrace His truths, and live in harmony with His principles and Him. Giving a breath of hope and doing life in God's way is right. Jesus Christ, the Son of God, gives you the experience with the God of love to know He is real and the only source of life, health, and happiness.

Addiction is a complex issue that not only affects the individual but also has a significant impact on relationships. The mental, emotional, and behavioral changes that often accompany addiction can strain even the strongest bonds. However, there is hope for healing and restoration. Couples and family counseling can provide a safe space to address the relational issues that have arisen as a result of addictive behaviors. We can cultivate relationships grounded in divine truths by acknowledging the importance of the love triangle of Science, Scripture, and Experience. Take the necessary steps to strengthen your connections and choose love over addiction.

---

[57] McMinn, M. R. (2011). Psychology, Theology, and Spirituality in Christian Counseling. Tyndale House Publishers.

The Bible Says...

"When the selfish nature is in charge, it is obvious, because the life reflects the destructive behaviors of the selfish nature,...All such behaviors destroy the image of God in humankind, dethrone reason, sear the conscience, inflame the debasing desires, and result in individuals—although created in God's image—digressing into nonthinking, animalistic brutes incapable of entering the kingdom of God." (Galatians 5:19-21 REM)

CHAPTER 7

UNMASKING THE BRAIN ON DRUGS

Before speaking of drugs and their effects on the brain, let us first gain a simplified understanding of brain development. The brain's makeup is that of neural developmental mechanisms. When there's a neuropsychiatric problem, issues can be traced back to deviations in the brain's neural development.

Some Neuropsychiatric disorders (Mental Health Disorders), such as schizophrenia (SZ), bipolar disorder (BD), generalized anxiety disorder (AD), major depressive disorder (MDD), and attention deficit hyperactivity disorder (ADHD), are increasingly common and can become highly impairing conditions.[58]

Consider this simple comparison. I'm sure there are many reasons for tree or plant trimming. However, one of the dominant reasons is maintaining the tree or plant health (vibrancy).

In the brain, "Exuberant Synaptogenesis" is the trimming or pruning of neurons during early brain development, from infancy to 3 years of age and ending at 20. Evidence suggests pruning may lightly continue through life. We have an astounding number of brain neurons during infancy and early childhood competing for dominance of such abilities as memory, learning, and other life processes. "Each neuron may be connected to up to 10,000 other neurons, passing

---

[58] Retrieved from https://www.ncbi.nlm.nih.gov/pmc/articles/PMC6551216/

signals to each other via as many as 1,000 trillion synapses." (Zhang, J., 2019)[59]

"Early synaptic pruning is mostly influenced by our genes. Later on, it's based on our experiences. In other words, whether or not a synapse is pruned is influenced by the experiences a developing child has with the world around them. Constant stimulation causes synapses to grow and become permanent. But if a child receives little stimulation the brain will keep fewer of those connections...According to newer research, synaptic pruning actually continues into early adulthood and stops sometime in the late 20s." (Cafasso 2018) [60]

As the brain initially develops, cells multiply, interact with one another, and grow more robust. Brain connections and neuron pruning are activity-dependent, like trimming a fruit tree.

Driven by activity and competition, the pruning of cells and neurons is regulated. The older and less used parts are discontinued to benefit the newer, more active components as the child and adolescent are stimulated through their activity, environment, parental attention, and parental-induced activity such as music, walking and talking, laughing and crying. The less active brain cells and neurons give way to the more active neural pathways.

Experience is the portal of fine-tuning neural connections. Thus, our stimulation directs us to be what we will be.

Similar but more subtle changes occur in adulthood during learning as neural plasticity manages synaptic connections and codes memories.

The negative impact of trauma, drugs, addictive behaviors, toxins, fear & apprehension are among the experiences that negatively change the brain. Abnormal experiences may permanently alter the patterns of those connections. Changes in regional brain activity that occur through repetition strengthen learning.

Individual neurons receive signals from thousands of neurons passing along messages. Particular bits of information travel to the

---

[59] Zhang, J. (2019) Basic Neural Units of the Brain: Neurons, Synapses and Action Potential. Retrieved from https://arxiv.org/abs/1906.01703

[60] Cafasso, J., (2018) What is Synaptic Pruning. https://www.healthline.com/health/synaptic-pruning#timeline] [https://www.pnas.org/doi/10.1073/pnas.1105108108

peripheral sensory neurons representing the ever-changing networks that shift participation from one network to another (such as limbic, executive, language, etc.). The sophistication of these networks depends on both neurons and their connections.

Some other brain regions will control speech, judgment, thinking and reasoning, problem-solving, emotions, and learning—other functions related to our senses of vision, hearing, touch, and smell.

Through our DNA, the shaping of neurons in common clusters is dictated by their function. Each group receives, processes, and transmits information. Each region has distinct functions. Each part also depends on the previous for the uninterrupted cycle of metabolic flow (blood, electrical, chemical) needed for thinking, planning, and behavior.

Dendrites receive signals from other neurons and convey these to the cell bodies. The cell body contains the genetic information for the necessary elements of cellular function. Over long distances, the Axon transmits information to terminals (neurons, muscles, and glands), or making contact with other neurons affects our cells, and the cycle reinitiates.

Chemical mediation occurs in most synaptic connections. Chemical synapses are slower than electrical ones but allow for signal amplification. The changes brought by intoxicating illicit drugs, alcohol, or intoxicating behaviors will change the flow and amplification of the synaptic connections.

A cascade of damage occurs to life and the brain when abusing alcohol, drugs, and addictive behaviors (repetitive harming behaviors) into brain mechanics.

The Bible says...

"...Therefore, keep your minds clear and sharp, and maintain governance of yourselves so that you can always talk clearly with God...Those who live with the selfish nature in charge have their minds bent on self-indulgence and selfish pursuits; but those who live in harmony with the Spirit of truth and love have their minds focused on living in harmony with God's principles of truth, love, and liberty. The mind of the selfish person is filled

with death, but the mind governed by the principles of the Spirit of truth and love is filled with life and peace."
(1 Peter 4:7b; Romans 8:5-6 REM)

THE BRAIN ON STIMULANTS — UNVEILING THE PROFOUND EFFECTS OF 'UPPERS' ON COGNITIVE FUNCTION AND BEYOND

To comprehensively understand the impact of drugs on brain function, it is essential to categorize the various substances based on their effects. For this purpose, we classify them into three distinct groups: stimulants (commonly referred to as 'uppers'), depressants ('downers'), and a third category encompassing substances with varied effects, known as 'all-a-rounders.' In our current discussion, the focus is on stimulants, or 'uppers,' and their specific impact on the brain.

What are Uppers?

Stimulants, or 'uppers,' are drugs that accelerate brain activity, leading to increased alertness, attention, and energy. They achieve this by boosting certain neurotransmitters in the brain, particularly dopamine and norepinephrine. These neurotransmitters are associated with heightened arousal, increased heart rate and blood pressure, and a general sense of euphoria or increased energy. However, the prolonged use of stimulants can lead to a variety of adverse effects on the brain, including addiction, altered brain function, and even cognitive deficits.

Uppers is a description used to explain the material that elevates the brain and body activity and is commonly known as "stimulants." Stimulants differ from very robust, such as cocaine and amphetamines, to weak ones, like caffeine and nicotine. However, nicotine is proven to cause the most severe long-term health problems.

Like a rocket launching, stimulants generate a chemical thrust, stimulating chemical compounds throughout the user's brain and body. The stimulation boosts the brain's reward and pleasure centers into intense action. Constricting blood vessels, racing heart rate, and hypertension come from using or abusing stimulants.

In his book, *Uppers, Downers, All-a-rounders*, Doctor of Pharmacology, Darryl S. Inaba (Inaba 2020)[61] identifies seven Central Nervous System (CNS) stimulants (uppers) as:

- Cocaine (hydrochloride, freebase, crack)
- Amphetamines (Adderall, "crystal" meth, speed)
- Amphetamine congeners [chemical substances related to amphetamines] (Ritalin, diet pills)
- Plan stimulants (khat, betel nuts, ephedra, Yohimbe), and look-alike stimulants
- Caffeine (coffee, tea, colas, energy drinks, chocolate)
- Nicotine (cigars, cigarettes, smokeless tobacco) and designer stimulants (bath salts)
- Psychostimulants (e.g., ecstasy and other phenylethylamines) can have psychedelic effects in addition to methamphetamine-like stimulatory ones.

Upper's Effects On The Brain

The use of stimulants triggers an electrical and chemical effect on the CNS. The brain signals the release of energy chemicals, hormones, and adrenaline neurotransmitters. Uppers disrupt the usual ebb and flow of chemicals, blood, and charged particles that energize muscles and maintain alertness and the 24-hour mind and body rhythm.

Sometimes, the body needs extra energy for exercising or during fear, sex, or battle. At these moments, the mind releases the above-described energy. Typically, the body absorbs the excess energy sources within minutes of the stimulating source.

However, adding uppers brings excess energy, short-circuiting the CNS (which consists of the brain and spinal cord).

---

61 Inaba, Darryl, et.al., (2020) <u>Uppers, Downers, All Arounders</u>, Eigth Edition, 732, CNS Publications Inc., Ashland, OR.

More potent stimulants such as methamphetamine and "crack" cocaine keep chemicals in circulation by blocking their reabsorption and metabolism, thus greatly exaggerating the stimulant effects. As this process continues for hours, even days, it supplies the body with an enormous amount of excess energy that needs to be released.

It is common for a "meth" abuser to stay high for three to five days without sleep, only to repeat the event several times.

When only taking uppers occasionally, the body has time to recover. Even with occasional use, stimulants can have a cascading effect that tears down the overall health of the brain, body, and identity.

Long-term, continuous, or heavy consumption of uppers depletes energy supplies and the body's reserves. As a result, the "crash" is followed by withdrawal symptoms (sometimes flu-like) and depression that last for days, weeks, and even months. Crash severity depends on the length of use, stimulant strength, degree of biochemical disturbance, and pre-existing mental or emotional problems.

Because tolerance occurs, the feel-good of the high significantly reduces over time. But, the fear of the crash becomes more significant than the void of intoxication leading to out-of-control abuse. During these periods of being out of control, many stimulant abusers lie, cheat, steal, and kill, even if it goes against their morality.

Stimulant users and abusers experience a disturbed mental and emotional state of mind. Enhancing and disrupting the normal brain flow of neurotransmitters increases self-confidence, produces euphoria, and makes the user feel omnipotent. However, continued use leads to a decline in mental performance and favorability. The user or abuser becomes more irritable, assertive, talkative, paranoid, restless, sleepless, and sometimes aggressive.

The unnatural use of stimulants gains energy and confidence by reducing the body's energy supply. Compare this to the natural replenishment of energy reserves through relaxation, sleep, daytime sleep, light morning exercises, prayer, rest, harmony, proper nutrition, and a healthy lifestyle. Natural methods are used to create energy reserves without allowing excess to build up.

Unorthodox methods of stimulant use deplete the body's energy reserves, requiring it to switch off to recover. The natural process always works. The abnormal form causes tolerance and psychological dependence to develop, so excessive use depletes the body's resources and can damage neurochemistry.

Dr. Inaba says, "If you want to speed up, slow down."

The Bible Says...

"So come to me, all who are tired, worn down and exhausted from fear, selfishness, and fighting to survive on your own, and I will give you rest. Join up with me and learn my methods—the principles upon which life is built to operate—for I am gentle and humble in heart, and you will find healing and rest for your souls. For joining up with me and living in harmony with the way life is designed to operate is what makes life easy and lightens life's burdens." (Matthew 11:28-30 REM)

The Brain on Sedatives Redefines Pain Relief and Restorative Bliss

Sedatives, also called downers, are used both for their medicinal properties of pain relief, cough suppression, and diarrhea control and for their psychological properties of sedation and euphoria. Prescription drug abuse is the leading cause of preventable deaths in the United States. Almost half of those 40,000 deaths are due to downers in the classification of tranquilizers such as opioid painkillers.

Unlike stimulants — uppers, which stimulate the central nervous system (CNS), depressants — downers — depress overall CNS function, resulting in sedation, muscle relaxation, drowsiness, and, if used in excess, coma. While stimulants release and amplify the body's natural stimulatory neurochemicals, sedatives induce a high or intoxication and often suppress impulses and emotions. At the same time, depressants exert their effects through various biochemical processes in different brain regions, the spinal cord, and other organs such as the heart.

There are four categories of sedatives/tranquilizers — downers, also called CNS depressants:

- Opiates and opioids: Opium, heroin, oxycodone (OxyContin), hydrocodone (Vicodin), buprenorphine (Suboxone), and methadone
- Sedative-hypnotics: benzodiazepines, including alprazolam (Xanax) and clonazepam (Klonopin); barbiturates such as butalbital; Z-hypnotics such as zolpidem (Ambient); and others like Ramelteon (Rozerem)
- Alcohol: beer, wine, and spirits
- Other: Antihistamines, skeletal muscle relaxants, and over-the-counter tranquilizers like sleeping pills.

Body Effects

Small doses of sedatives depress the CNS, which slows the heart and breathing rates, relaxes muscles, impairs coordination, induces sleep, dulls the senses, relieves pain, and controls diarrhea. Opiates and opioids can cause nausea, constriction of the pupils, and constipation.

Excessive consumption of alcohol and tranquilizers, sleeping pills, or opioids can impair physical coordination, cause slurred speech, cause digestive problems, cause sexual dysfunction, and cause tissue dependence.

High doses or in combination with other sedatives can result in dangerous respiratory depression, overdose, and coma.

Mental and Emotional Effects

Initially, small doses (especially alcohol) act as stimulants — uppers — as they reduce stiffness, which can lead to loose and sometimes irresponsible behavior.

When taking more of the drug, the general depressive effects predominate, relaxing and numbing the mind, reducing anxiety, and controlling some neuroses. Some sedatives can also induce euphoria or a sense of well-being.

Long-term use of tranquilizers can lead to psychological and physical dependence and addiction. Because of their potentially lower overdose potential, benzodiazepines dominated the prescription tranquilizer market for some time. Prescription drug abuse had spread to all sections of society by the year 2000.

A significant example of the deteriorating effect of alcohol's long-term use/abuse was recently published. Researchers assessed dementia risk based on two-year changes in alcohol consumption among approximately 4 million people in South Korea. After about seven years, the light drinker was 21% less likely to have dementia, and the moderate drinker was 17% less likely to have it. Heavy drinking was associated with an 8% increase in risk (JAMA 2023).[62]

Cross tolerance is when a person develops an ability to tolerate one drug and other drugs of the same classification, such as alcohol and opioids. For example, a heroin addict will endure morphine, methadone, etc., even if the addict has never taken them before. The exact biological mechanisms that produce tolerance to one opioid also make tolerance to others.

Tissue dependence occurs due to the body's biological adaptation to long-term drug use. The body compensates by restoring homeostatic levels and altering homeostatic components to withstand chemical stressors. The reset creates processes by which the body responds to chemical stressors to compensate for biological stability during prolonged drug exposure. Changes can be extensive, especially with the use of sedatives. The tissue addiction returns faster with each relapse of the offender.

Since alcohol has been the most popular sedative — downer — for many years, the following video will focus on alcohol and a possible key factor in creating an addictive personality.

---

[62] Retrieved from *JAMA Netw Open*. 2023;6(2):e2254771. doi:10.1001/jamanetworkopen.2022.54771 https://jamanetwork.com/journals/jamanetworkopen/fullarticle/2800994

The Bible Says...

"Therefore, surrender yourselves under God's almighty healing hand that he might restore you, uplifting you to his ideal in due time. Pour out all your worries, frustrations and burdens upon him, because he cares for you. Stay calm and keep a clear head: do not allow your emotions to take charge, because Satan, your enemy, is stalking around, roaring like a lion, seeking to consume you with fear and doubt. But resist him and don't be afraid; keep your trust in God strong, because you know that your fellow believers throughout the world are also being attacked in the same way."

"For God did not give you a character of insecurity, doubt and fear, but a mind and character of confidence, power in the truth, love, and self-control."

(1 Peter 5:6-9; 2 Timothy 1:7 REM)

CHAPTER 8

THE COMPLEX INTERPLAY OF ALCOHOL, DRUGS, AND THE BRAIN — A DEEP DIVE INTO CO-USAGE PATTERNS AND THEIR IMPACT ON MENTAL AND PHYSICAL HEALTH

Alcohol use and abuse are often with many other psychoactive drugs to enhance, counteract, or modify the effects of different substances and behaviors. In one study, 80% of participants used alcohol and marijuana together, and up to 70% smoked cigarettes and drank alcohol.

Highs like cocaine or methamphetamine and alcohol together form a "speedball" to counteract the depression that chronic alcohol use can cause.

Using alcohol alters mood or state of mind. It is a depressant, so the incidence of depression in heavy drinkers (often caused by alcohol) is five times higher than in the average population.

Anxiety is a condition more than twice as typical in heavy drinkers. Pre-existing mental health problems must be treated concurrently with alcoholism to avoid relapse.

Symptoms of alcoholism can be confused with or masked by those of particular mental, mood, and personality disorders.

Fetal damage during pregnancy due to fetal alcohol syndrome (FAS) and other fetal alcohol spectrum disorders (FASD) is typical.

A pregnant woman's lifestyle, use, or drinking can affect the fetus as much as alcohol or drugs.

It can take three months to 30 years before alcoholism develops, so drinkers must assess their current level of use and susceptibility to compulsive use.

For thousands of years, humans have adapted to alcohol and developed a culture of drinking and addiction. The long history with alcohol brings us to the question: "Is alcohol abuse a significant factor in overall addiction?"

The Catalyst For Alcoholism and Addictions

Alcohol, made up of ethanol, can be considered a toxin or poison to the body. The body's initial reaction to high concentrations of ethanol intake is a burning sensation as it travels down the esophagus.

Alarms go off when ethanol enters the body's primary filtration system, the liver, to break down harmful substances. During liver processing, ethanol converts to less toxic acetaldehyde. However, acetaldehyde, still a toxin, is a significant cause of "hangover" symptoms and causes other significant side effects during alcohol consumption.

About 5 to 10 minutes after consuming alcohol, the drinker may feel the effects of a severe hangover for 30 minutes to several hours. Symptoms include flushed skin, increased heart rate, shortness of breath, nausea, vomiting, throbbing headache, blurred vision, confusion, fainting/loss of consciousness, and circulatory collapse. Further processing is required to break down acetaldehyde into acetaldehyde dehydrogenase (AD).

Acetaldehyde does not completely degrade in the liver due to genetic interference in the form of the A1 allele gene. Alleles are linked genes that help determine traits such as hair color, eye color, height, weight, etc.

In a landmark study, the A1 allele of the dopamine D2 receptor gene was the first gene identified as a cause of addiction, discovered in 1990 by researchers Ernest Noble and Kenneth Blum (Inaba 2020). Their study found a very high incidence of this gene in severe alcoholics.

Subsequent studies have shown that this gene is also associated with drug addiction and addictive behaviors. [63]

Dominant traits and alleles usually refer to the inheritance of attributes passed vertically from parent to child. The feature or disorder associated with that gene affects both parent and child. The most common form is autosomal dominant, where the related gene is located on one of 22 non-sex chromosomes, and affected individuals have two alleles of the gene (one pathogenic and one benign). In this inheritance pattern, carrying one pathogenic allele is enough to confer the trait on the person. Then, an affected individual with only one of her two copies of the virulence gene has a 50% chance of passing the marker on to their offspring (Biesecker 2023).[64]

Noble & Blum found that the marker gene was only present in 19-21% of non-alcoholic, non-addictive, and non-obsessive individuals but is over-represented in:

- 69% of alcoholic subjects
- 45% of compulsive overeaters
- 48% of smokers
- 52% of cocaine addicts
- 51% of pathological gamblers
- 76% of pathological gamblers with drug problems
- 45% of people with Tourette's syndrome (compulsive verbal outbursts or muscular tics)
- 49% of ADHD compared to 27% of a control group

Allele frequency indicates how often an allele occurs within a population. You determine the frequency by counting the frequency with which the allele occurs within the population and dividing by the total number of gene copies.

Evidence is accumulating that alcohol consumption can increase levels of acetaldehyde (AcH) derivatives in the brain, which may be of

---

[63] Ibid. Inaba, (2020)

[64] Biesecker, L. (2023) Retrieved from https://www.genome.gov/genetics-glossary/Dominant-Traits-and-Alleles

pharmacological importance (Deng and Deitrich 2008).[65] The study suggests that AcH itself has reinforcing properties, which could imply that some of the behavioral and pharmacological effects attributed to ethanol might be due to the formation of AcH, supporting its involvement in ethanol addiction —it is accumulating in the brain taking longer (years) to dissipate during abstinence.

Epigenetics

The biblical principle from 1 Corinthians 15:33 (NIV), *"Do not be misled: 'Bad company corrupts good character,'"* underscores the profound impact of our associations on our moral and ethical development. This concept can also be extended to neurology, where detrimental influences within or among neural networks can compromise healthy brain development. Just as negative associations can deteriorate one's character, similarly, unfavorable environments can hinder the optimal growth and functionality of brain cells.

The human brain is constantly changing. Not only do life experiences change the circuits in our brains, but new research also shows that life experiences change gene expression, passing to our children.

Epigenetics studies how cells control gene activity without altering their DNA sequences. "Epi" is Greek for "more than," and "epigenetic" describes factors beyond the genetic code. Epigenetic changes (demethylation and methylation) to DNA control whether a gene is turned on or off. These modifications are added to the DNA and do not alter the sequence of the DNA building blocks.

Each cell expresses or turns on only some of its genes at any time. The remaining genes are repressed or turned off. The process of turning genes on and off is called gene regulation.

Gene regulation is an integral part of normal development. During development, genes are switched on and off in different patterns, so

---

[65] Deng, X.-s., et al. (2008). Putative role of brain acetaldehyde in ethanol addiction. Current Drug Abuse Reviews, 1(1), 3-8.

brain cells, for example, look and behave differently than liver or muscle cells. Gene regulation also enables cells to respond rapidly to environmental changes.

More often, gene regulation occurs during transcription — copying RNA from DNA. During transcription, ribonucleic acid (RNA) polymerase makes copies of genes from DNA to mRNA as needed. In molecular biology, messenger ribonucleic acid (mRNA) is a single-stranded RNA molecule corresponding to a gene sequence of a gene and ribosomes in protein synthesis interpretation.

Transcription factors are proteins activated by environmental signals. These proteins bind to the regulatory regions of the gene, increasing or decreasing the transcription level. By controlling the transcription level, this process can determine when and how much of a protein product the genome produces.

Epigenetic modification patterns differ between individuals, within different tissues, and even within other cells within a tissue. Environmental influences such as diet and exposure to pollutants can affect the library of records within each cell — epigenome. Epigenetic modifications are maintained from cell to cell as cells divide and, sometimes, are passed on through generations (NIH 2021).[66]

"I lay the sins of the parents upon their children and grandchildren; the entire family is affected—even children in the third and fourth generations." (Exodus 34:6-7 NLT)

Understanding this gives us insight into how habits are formed and broken. Constant engagement with specific behavioral patterns activates the same circuits that cause changes in DNA that produce proteins that strengthen the particular brain circuits that correspond to the behavior. Conversely, DNA expression changes when behavior ceases, and the circuitry remains idle, causing the brain circuits to revert over time.

"Therefore with all my heart I urge you, brothers and sisters, to consider how merciful God is in providing his Remedy, and to surrender your entire being to God as a living sacrifice — to be healed and transformed into

---

[66] NIH (2021) https://medlineplus.gov/genetics/understanding/howgeneswork/epigenome/

God's image. This is the most reasonable, logical and intelligent worship you could ever offer. Do not continue to practice the destructive methods of selfishness, which infect the world, but be completely transformed into God's image by the renewing of your mind. Then you will value God's principles, practice his methods, and discern his will—his good, pleasing and perfect will." (Romans 12:1-2 REM)

CHAPTER 9

ALCOHOLISM AND THE
ADDICTIVE PERSONALITY

What Causes The Addictive
Personality And Alcoholism?

Addictive personality is a concept that refers to a set of personality traits that may make an individual more susceptible to developing addictions. This concept, while popular in lay discussions, is not a formal psychiatric diagnosis. It's important to note that addiction is a complex condition influenced by a complex interplay of genetic, neurobiological, psychological, social, environmental, and spiritual factors. It's essential to approach this topic with an understanding of this complexity and the nuances involved in addiction research.

Genetics plays a significant role in addiction. Studies have shown that genetics account for about half of the likelihood that an individual will develop an addiction. This genetic predisposition can be linked to impulsivity and reward-seeking behavior (Agrawal 2008).[67]

What causes addiction is an important issue. In 1970, Davis and Walsh published ideas that challenged existing theories about

---

[67] Agrawal, A., & Lynskey, M. T. (2008). The genetic epidemiology of cannabis use, abuse and dependence. Addiction, 103(6), 787-809.

alcoholism and stimulated research to produce some intriguing new concepts about alcoholism and addiction (Cotman 1980).[68]

Davis and Walsh argued that alcohol derivatives promote the formation of compounds with opiate-like properties in the brain. Once dopamine metabolizes, conversion to dopaldehyde requires further cleavage by aldehyde dehydrogenase. Aldehyde dehydrogenase is also necessary to form acetaldehyde, the first product of alcohol metabolism. Not all dopaldehyde is metabolized in the body because the enzymes prefer acetaldehyde. At high concentrations, dopaldehyde condenses to form tetrahydropapaveroline (THP), a benzyl-tetrahydroisoquinoline alkaloid derivative of dopamine. THP is a precursor of the opium alkaloids found in poppies and is more addictive than morphine (CT 2010).[69]

"Twin studies have already identified a genetic connection to alcoholism and other drug addictions. Other twin studies have shown a connection between heredity and other compulsive behaviors which don't involve psychoactive drugs." (Inaba 2020)[70]

A process called switching (PBS)[71] turns genes on and off. Feeding different nutrients to a control group of genetically identical mice produces different coat colors in their offspring. However, they remain genetically similar. The switching on or off particular genes depends on introducing a specific methyl group. Taking cocaine turns on chains previously switched off. As a result, increased protein causes a higher craving for more and more illicit substances. The person's future children are likelier to be born with a high propensity for addiction (NIH 2021).[72]

Gene regulation, a vital aspect of normal cellular function and development, involves the selective expression of specific genes at various

---

[68] Cotman, C. & McGaugh, J., "Mechanisms of Physical Dependence, Tolerance and Withdrawal" in Behavioral Neuroscience, 1980

[69] Comprehensive Toxicology (Second Edition) Volume 1, 2010, Pages 411-445 https://www.sciencedirect.com/topics/neuroscience/tetrahydropapaveroline

[70] Inaba, 732

[71] PBS & WGBH Educational Foundation. (2023) https://gpb.pbslearningmedia.org/resource/novat10.sci.life.evo.fruitfly/switching-genes-on-and-off/

[72] NIH (2021) https://medlineplus.gov/genetics/understanding/howgeneswork/geneonoff/

times. Only a portion of a cell's genes are active at any given moment, while the remaining genes remain suppressed. This dynamic process, essential for life, is intricate and needs to be fully comprehended.

During development, gene regulation is crucial in differentiating cells into various types, such as brain, liver, or muscle cells, by controlling gene activity in diverse patterns. Moreover, this regulatory mechanism equips cells to adapt swiftly to environmental changes.

The modulation of gene expression predominantly occurs during transcription, the phase where DNA information is transferred to mRNA. Environmental cues or signals from other cells activate transcription factors, proteins that bind to a gene's regulatory regions, thus influencing the transcription level. This regulation of transcription dictates the timing and quantity of protein a gene produces (Lodish 2000).[73]

Alcoholism and opiate addiction are closely linked through common biochemical pathways.

Certain neurobiological factors, such as the functioning of the brain's reward system, are believed to contribute to addictive behaviors. People with specific neurotransmitter imbalances or brain structure differences may be more prone to addiction (Volkow 2015).[74]

Addiction research boils down to thousands of years of alcohol abuse, chemically altering the human brain, making it more susceptible to addiction to stimulants, tranquilizers, and hallucinogens.

However, there is a broader perspective to recognize. Addiction models include the addictive disease model (medical model), behavioral/environmental model, academic model, and predisposing stress theories of addiction.

This article focuses primarily on the academic model of addiction. In this model, addiction occurs when the body adapts to the toxic effects of drugs at the biochemical and cellular level in a process called allostasis –- the stress-induced restoration of balance.

---

[73] Lodish, H., Berk, A., Zipursky, S. L., Matsudaira, P., Baltimore, D., & Darnell, J. (2000). In their work, "Molecular Cell Biology" (4th ed.), New York: W. H. Freeman
[74] Volkow, N. D., & Morales, M. (2015). The brain on drugs: from reward to addiction. Cell, 162(4), 712-725.

When you take enough drugs long enough, your body and brain as protective mechanisms change and adapt. This attempt to restore balance creates long-lasting changes that lead to and reinforce addictions. Another addiction model is the predisposing stress theory of addiction. This model unifies the theory and views addiction as a process that spans the user's life from birth to death. A predisposition is a constitutional predisposition or predisposition to develop a particular disorder under certain conditions.

Predisposition (diathesis) to addiction results from genetic and environmental influences (e.g., childhood abuse, family drug use, or destructive behavior). Chemical groups called methyl groups are attached to DNA regions to modify gene expression during a lifetime. Also, returning to typical behavior becomes difficult due to changes in brain chemistry, brain function, and even the presentation of new epigenetic genes (Inaba 2020).[75]

Personality traits such as impulsivity, sensation-seeking, and a high need for excitement and novelty are often associated with addictive personality and behaviors. Mental health issues like depression and anxiety can also increase the risk of developing an addiction (Zilberman 2003).[76]

Environment plays a crucial role in the development of addictive personality and behaviors. This includes factors like exposure to drugs or alcohol at a young age, peer pressure, stress, and trauma (Hawkins 1992).[77]

Early life experiences, including parenting styles and childhood trauma, can influence the development of traits associated with addictive personality and behaviors (Anda 2006).[78]

---

[75] Inaba, (2020) 81-84

[76] Zilberman, M. L., Tavares, H., & el-Guebaly, N. (2003). Gender similarities and differences: the prevalence and course of alcohol- and other substance-related disorders. Journal of Addictive Diseases, 22(Suppl 1), 61-74.

[77] Hawkins, J. D., Catalano, R. F., & Miller, J. Y. (1992). Risk and protective factors for alcohol and other drug problems in adolescence and early adulthood: implications for substance abuse prevention. Psychological Bulletin, 112(1), 64-105.

[78] Anda, R. F., Felitti, V. J., Bremner, J. D., Walker, J. D., Whitfield, C., Perry, B. D., ... & Giles, W. H. (2006). The enduring effects of abuse and related adverse experiences in childhood. European Archives of Psychiatry and Clinical Neuroscience, 256(3), 174-186.

The Spiritual Aspect of the Addictive Personality: *The Absence of Modeling Love!*

We have known for years that addiction runs in families. In other words, the more ancestry of addiction, the higher the risk of developing addiction problems. Parents are passing along changes in gene expression (Epigenetics) to the next generation. God's omniscience engineers our bodies to inherit our parent's goodness and badness. Which is it going to be for your child?

Our Father God created our gene structure with the ability to adapt and change based on our choices and experiences. When we choose unhealthy thoughts and behaviors, we change our epigenetic instructions and pass those changes on to our children — turning sets of DNA on or off. Mentally and emotionally, the result can be the formation of an addictive personality.

God warned that those opposed to His truths could experience adverse consequences passed down to three or four generations of their family, while those who know and love Him will experience His love.

"You must not make for yourself an idol of any kind or an image of anything in the heavens or on the earth or in the sea. You must not bow down to them or worship them, for I, the Lord your God, am a jealous God who will not tolerate your affection for any other Gods. I lay the sins of the parents upon their children; the entire family is affected—even children in the third and fourth generations of those who reject me. But I lavish unfailing love for a thousand generations on those who love me and obey my commands." (Exodus 20:4-6 NLT)

If it is true that groups of DNA are turned on and off (gene regulation), are we responsible for the handed-down effect on our generations? The medical model of addiction gives scientific evidence that what parents are, to a great extent, so will the children be.

The parent's physical condition, temperament, appetite, and mental and moral inclinations will likely be reproduced in the child.

The more unselfish parents' goals are, the higher their spiritual, mental, and physical talents, and the better equipped the child will be. By nurturing the best in themselves, parents exert influence to shape society and improve future generations.

When playing with addictive behaviors and substances, the parent's energy becomes wasted, and millions are ruined now and in the future. Parents are to help their children resist these life-destroying temptations through modeling. Preparations must begin before a child is born so that they can successfully fight the negatively seducing world influences giving way to addictions.

The mother and father nourish the child through a lifeline of love, building the child's physical health while exerting a mental and spiritual influence to shape the mind and character.

God's promises are contingent on the absence of false gods (idols). In other words, we must return to the truth about God. I believe worshiping the God of Love strengthens the higher cortex and calms the limbic system. But all the wrong notions of God activate the limbic system (basement) and do not heal the higher cortex (upper room).

Andrew Newberg is a neuroscientist known for his research on the neurological basis of religious and spiritual experiences. In his book How God Changes Your Brain, he discusses how different spiritual practices, including meditation and prayer, can affect the brain (2009).[79]

A study investigating the brain regions involved in personal prayer suggests that areas related to social interaction and empathy are engaged during this process (Schjoedt, U. 2009).[80]

The study by Beauregard and Paquette (2006) aimed to explore the neural correlates of mystical experiences, particularly in intense religious or spiritual feelings. This research was conducted with a group of Carmelite nuns known for their deep spiritual practices. The key focus was identifying specific brain regions activated during their self-reported mystical experiences.[81]

---

[79] Newberg, A. B., & Waldman, M. R. (2009). How God changes your brain: Breakthrough findings from a leading neuroscientist. New York, NY: Ballantine Books.
[80] Schjoedt, U., Stødkilde-Jørgensen, H., Geertz, A. W., & Roepstorff, A. (2009). Highly religious participants recruit areas of social cognition in personal prayer. *Social Cognitive and Affective Neuroscience, 4*(3), 199-207. https://doi.org/10.1093/scan/nsn050
[81] Beauregard, M., & Paquette, V. (2006). Neural correlates of a mystical experience in Carmelite nuns. *Neuroscience Letters, 405*(3), 186-190. https://doi.org/10.1016/j.neulet.2006.06.060.

The methodology involved using functional magnetic resonance imaging (fMRI) to monitor brain activity in these nuns. During the scanning process, the nuns were asked to recall and relive their most profound mystical experiences, which they had previously reported as feelings of union with the divine. The researchers compared the brain imaging data obtained during these recollections to the nuns' brain activity during ordinary resting states.

The study found that several brain regions were significantly activated during the mystical experiences. These areas included concentration, self-consciousness, emotion, and body representation. The activation of these regions suggested that mystical experiences, at least in this context, could be associated with specific neural activities.

Within the Brain's "Upper room," the anterior frontal lobe, specifically the prefrontal cortex, plays a crucial role in what might be considered "good thinking." It encompasses various aspects of cognitive function, such as decision-making, problem-solving, and planning.

The dorsolateral prefrontal cortex (DLPFC) is particularly significant in decision-making, planning, and working memory. It integrates sensory and mnemonic information and regulates intellectual function and action —right, good, and loving thinking.

The ventromedial prefrontal cortex (VMPFC) is involved in the processing of risk and fear, and it plays a role in regulating emotions, empathy, and social cognition, which are essential for what might be considered 'good' or 'wise' decision-making.

The anterior cingulate cortex (ACC), part of the frontal lobe, is involved in functions like error detection, task anticipation, motivation, and modulation of emotional responses. It contributes to cognitive flexibility and problem-solving skills.

The region of the Orbitofrontal Cortex is involved in processing rewards and punishments and is also crucial in decision-making, especially in socially complex situations.

The functionality of the prefrontal cortex is not isolated; it works in conjunction with other parts of the brain. Integrating its activities with other neural regions leads to complex cognitive behaviors often called "good thinking." It's also important to note that individual differences, such as genetics, environmental factors, and educational background, can influence the functioning of these brain regions (Kandel 2013).[82]

These "good thinking" regions of the "upper room" can be seen as opposed to the brain's limbic system, which is guided by the Amygdala's threat alarm. Fear and apprehension, self-protection, selfishness, bitterness, and depression are foundational characteristics of the addictive personality dwelling in the brain's dark basement. PET Scans have demonstrated that when the upper room's DLPFC is active, the basement's Amygdala must deactivate, and vice versa.

These studies and others give evidence of an interrelationship between love, fear, and the addictive personality. *"There is no fear in love. But perfect love drives out fear because fear has to do with punishment. The one who fears is not made perfect in love."* (1 John 4:18 NIV)

In the realm of love, dread finds no place to reside, for love, in its most complete and mature form, can dispel fear. This is because fear is often entangled with the anticipation of divine retribution. Therefore, an individual who harbors fear, particularly in the context of God's judgment, has not yet fully grasped the depth and breadth of God's love. A reciprocal relationship exists between love and fear; they live in a delicate balance where the presence of one diminishes the other. As love flourishes, fear recedes; conversely, love decreases when fear intensifies.

When gripped by fear, we become hypersensitive to real and perceived threats, prompting us to take measures we believe will safeguard us. This approach, however, needs to be directed more. Rather than embarking on an introspective journey to address and remedy our character flaws, fear causes us to focus predominantly on self-preservation. This outward focus often leads to wrongly attributing our failings to others (projection), which fosters division and erodes our love for our fellow human beings, characteristic of the addictive personality.

It is crucial, therefore, to cultivate complete and mature love, as this serves as a bulwark against the encroachment of fear and its accompanying consequences.

---

[82] Kandel, E. R., Schwartz, J. H., Jessell, T. M., Siegelbaum, S. A., Hudspeth, A. J., & Mack, S. (2013). *Principles of Neural Science* (5th ed.). McGraw-Hill Education.

The Bible Says...

"Some say: 'I am free to do everything'—but not everything is healthy. I am free to do everything, but I will not do anything that destroys my autonomy and takes away my freedom…Don't you comprehend what is happening? Your brain and body are designed as a complete unit to be a sacred temple for the Holy Spirit who comes from God and lives within you—intimately, in a bond of sacred love. You are not a self-originating or self-sustaining being: you belong in intimate connection with God! It cost God an infinite price to restore this connection with you, so let God and his love be revealed in the way you treat your body."

(1 Corinthians 6:12, 19-20 REM)

CHAPTER 10

UNMASKING RECOVERY —
THE CHALLENGES!

Are substance abuse and addiction treatments effective? Research-based addiction treatment typically reduces substance abuse by 40% to 60%. These rates are comparable to adherence rates observed in managing other chronic diseases such as asthma, hypertension, and diabetes. Addiction treatment dramatically reduces the unwanted consequences of family breakups, unemployment, criminal activity, or infectious diseases.

In the USA, daily, 1,740 die from a substance use disorder (SUD) or related cause; that's more than one death per minute. Between 35% and 40% of all hospital admissions are related to health problems caused by nicotine. 25% of all hospital admissions are related to alcohol-related health problems (Cotman 1980).[83]

These numbers are staggering compared to other serious health problems such as sexually transmitted diseases, liver disease, prostate or breast cancer, and stroke. Many of these diseases are often the result of substance abuse and addiction.

Substance abuse also profoundly impacts social systems, family relationships, crime, violence, mental health, and daily life. Reducing the effects of addiction will significantly improve the quality of life worldwide.

---

[83] Ibid. Cotman (1980)

Challenges of Addiction Treatment

Over the past several years, research, clinical practice, and discussion have identified eight principal elements of treating chemical and behavioral addictions (Inaba 2020)[84]

1. Medications
2. Imaging Systems
3. New Questionnaires & Techniques
4. Neuroscience
5. Evidence-based Practices
6. Coerced Treatment
7. Funding
8. Abstinence vs. Harm Reduction

MEDICATIONS: Drugs are more commonly used to treat addictions. As the use of addictive substances changes the chemical makeup of the brain, the search for drugs that lessen the effects of these chemical and structural changes continues. Here are some examples:

- Drugs to lessen withdrawal symptoms
- Drugs to lessen craving
- Substitute medications that are less damaging than the primary substance of abuse.
- Nutritional supplements
- Antidepressants

IMAGING SYSTEMS: Researchers use modern imaging systems and diagnostic techniques to visualize addiction's structural and physiological effects on the human brain. It is no longer accessible to deny having an addiction with the advent of sophisticated imaging techniques, genetic identification techniques, and sensitive neurochemical measurements. Due to indisputable physical indicators, behavioral disorders such as compulsions are more accessible to determine.

---

[84] Ibid. Inaba, (2020) 438-452

New imaging techniques can identify several brain circuit systems involved in addiction, such as survival/reward, motivation, memory/ learning, and control, easily observed through visualizing changes. They are most common in imaging studies of central nervous system (CNS) changes.

- CAT (Computerized Axial Tomography) scan uses X-rays to show structural changes in brain tissue due to medication.

- MRI (Magnetic Resonance Imaging) uses the positioning of magnetic cores to produce highly detailed 2D and 3D images of brain structures that reveal subtle changes in brain tissue caused by the use of psychotropic drugs, as well as brain abnormalities that indicate a propensity for substance abuse clues; for example, a smaller prefrontal cortex (11% smaller on average) found in people prone to anger and violence.

- fMRI (Functional MRI) is an MRI technique that provides information about brain metabolism. While performing the test, fMRI tracts work in different brain parts. Whereas MRI only offers structural information about the brain and how drugs affect brain structure over time, fMRI provides information about how the brain is affected by substance use disorders. It provides both functional and structural information.

- PET (Positron Emission Tomography) scans use the metabolism of radioactively labeled chemicals injected into the bloodstream to measure glucose metabolism, blood flow, oxygenation, and the naturally occurring neurotransmission affected by drugs. Visualize the effects of matter.

- SPECT scans (single-photon emission computed tomography) also use radio-tracers to measure cerebral blood flow and trigger metabolism to help determine whether the brain functions while on drugs. They are similar to PET scans but cheaper and easier to use.

- DTI (Diffusion Tensor Imaging) is an MRI technique that can provide information about connections between brain regions. It visualizes the pathways of nerve fibers through the brain's white matter and shows how parts of the brain interact with each other (e.g., the survival/reinforcement circuitry that communicates with the control areas of the addiction pathway).

According to Dr. Daniel Amen, M.D., founder of the Amen Clinic for Behavioral Medicine, "There's so much these scans and images of the brain can offer the field of addiction. We can show children, teenagers, and adults that drugs impact their brains. It's much more powerful than showing them a picture of Fried eggs and bacon. It's constructive when confronting denial to sit in front of a computer screen with somebody who has been using drugs, and they say, 'Oh, there are no problems.' And you say, 'Let's look at yours.' And it has turned many people around." (Inaba 2020)[85]

NEW QUESTIONNAIRES & TECHNIQUES: Experts in the field have developed new questionnaires and methods to objectively identify and assess the severity of alcohol and other substance abuse behaviors. This validated dozens of diagnostic tools. Tools range from simple 4-item self-report instruments such as the CAGE-AID test to the comprehensive 200-point Addiction/Alcohol Severity Index. Valid diagnostic criteria are now critical to matching patients to the appropriate level of therapeutic intervention, maximizing the limited resources available while yielding better outcomes. The most widely used and practical in toxicology is the Patient Placement Criteria of the American Society of Poisoning Medicine (ASAM PPC). The growing number of diagnostic tools for substance use disorders, coupled with the increasing acceptance of assessment tools for determining the severity of withdrawal symptoms, provides a guide to medical detoxification treatment.

NEUROSCIENCE: As neuroscience research advances, so does our understanding and appreciation of relapse and recovery. In 2005, scientists found decreased activity in five separate areas of our brain's neocortex, correlating it with a higher risk of relapse

---

[85] Ibid, Inaba, (2020), 440

in methamphetamine addicts who completed 28 days of inpatient treatment. Depending on the survival/enhancement circuits in the 'old brain' and the prefrontal cortex control circuits that drive people to substance abuse and block their ability to quit, brain differences also affect their ability to maintain sobriety.

Neocortical damage from methamphetamine use and abuse is an essential link between a person's will to live and their personality. The neocortex also plays an influential role in sleep, memory, and learning processes. In the neocortex, sensory information impairment contributes to personality changes, cognitive decline, and the progressive symptoms of neurodegenerative diseases such as dementia.

Next time, we'll look at evidence-based practices, coerced treatment, funding, and abstinence vs. harm reduction.

The Bible Says...

"Be vigilant in your lifestyle—make choices that are healthy and wise, not unhealthy and foolish— and make the most of every opportunity for growth, because the days in which we live are filled with temptations that lead to self-destruction. Don't be foolish, but understand God's methods and what he is trying to accomplish, so that you can cooperate intelligently with him. Do not get drunk on wine or get high on drugs, as it leads to wild living and destroys the brain. Instead, be filled with the Spirit of truth and love. When talking with each other, talk of God's love and character, and sing songs of praise together. Keep your hearts in tune with the Lord, and be thankful to God the Father for everything revealed in the character of our Lord Jesus Christ." (Ephesians 5:15-20 REM)

EVIDENCE-BASED PRACTICES AND FUNDING

In discussing addiction treatment's challenges, we have canvassed medications, imaging systems, new questionnaires & techniques, and neuroscience. We will discuss evidence-based practices, coerced treatment, funding, and abstinence vs. harm reduction.

Substance Use Disorder SUD, A Public Health Crisis

According to the National Institute of Drug Abuse (NIH), after decades of research, addiction is now understood to be a chronic, treatable brain disorder from which one can recover. Unfortunately, the rates of SUDs are climbing, as evidenced in 2022:[86]

- 20.4 million people in the United States were diagnosed with SUD in the past year
- Only 10.3 percent of people with past-year SUD received SUD treatment
- Nearly 71,000 people died of drug overdoses in 2019

Broad Spectrum of Treatment Initiatives

- **Fundamental Neuroscience:** Understanding how drugs affect the cells and circuits of the brain, how addiction occurs, and how genes and environment affect the brain
- **Epidemiology:** Monitoring emerging trends in drug use
- **Risk and Protective Factors:** Identifying the factors that influence drug use, addiction, access to care, and related health outcomes
- **Prevention:** Developing and testing approaches to mitigate risk factors, promote resilience, and prevent drug use, addiction, and their consequences
- **Treatment:** Developing and testing medications, devices, and behavioral therapies for addiction and its consequences
- **Implementation:** Optimizing approaches for scaling up and enhancing access to evidence-based treatment and prevention strategies

---

[86] https://nida.nih.gov/about-nida/legislative-activities/budget-information/fiscal-year-2022-budget-information-congressional-justification-national-institute-drug-abuse/ic-fact-sheet-2022

EVIDENCE BASED PRACTICES· What are the best practices in treatment? Should treatment practices be identical to be called a treatment program? What kind of evidence is needed, and how much?

In his 8th Edition book, "Uppers, Downers, All-a-rounders," Dr. Craig Inaba writes, "There is a greater emphasis on evidence-based best practices in treatment and a diminished appreciation of practice-based clinical management."[87]

The overall goal of any evidence-based approach is to maximize the likelihood that treatment will consistently produce positive outcomes.

Although convenient, identifying a good or five-star treatment service or program is more challenging than looking up reviews on a computer. Evidence-based practices aim to provide efficient treatment services.

Addiction researchers are working to bridge the gap between research results and clinical practice. Some possibilities guide the identification, implementation, and maintenance of evidence-based practices.

There is no general agreement on what comprises or fully supports evidence-based practice. It is improbable that there will ever be a single best treatment for substance abuse for all patients.

The University of Iowa established the Practice Improvement Collaborative (PIC) network to introduce evidence-based addiction services. The PIC is developing plans to ensure that community-based treatment facilities adopt evidence-based practices.

The Iowa PIC developed 13-point criteria[88] to operationalize evidence-based criteria:

1. At least one randomized clinical trial has shown this practice to be effective.
2. The practice has demonstrated effectiveness in several replicated research studies using different samples, at least one of which is comparable to the treatment population of our region or agency.

---

[87] Inaba, Craig, (2014) "Uppers, Downers, All-a-rounders," 8th Edition, p440, CNS Publications, Ashland, OR

[88] https://icsa.uiowa.edu/sites/icsa.uiowa.edu/files/projects/Evidence-Based Practices - Implementation Guide.pdf

3. The practice either targets behaviors or shows a good effect on behaviors that are generally accepted outcomes.

4. The practice can logistically be applied in rural and low-population-density areas in our region.

5. The practice is feasible: it can be used in a group format, is attractive to third-party payers, is low-cost, and training is available.

6. The practice is manualized or sufficiently operationalized for staff use. Its key components are laid out.

7. Providers and clients will accept the practice.

8. The practice is based on a clear and well-articulated theory.

9. The practice has associated methods of ensuring fidelity — and trust.

10. The practice can be evaluated.

11. The practice shows reasonable retention rates for clients.

12. The practice addresses cultural diversity and different populations.

13. The practice can be used by staff with diverse backgrounds and training.

COERCED TREATMENT: More than 70,000 addicts receive treatment in the 50 states that operate drug court programs. The criminal justice system sanctions involuntary/court-ordered (coerced) treatment by drug courts, mandatory convictions, probation/probation rules, and state or federal laws mandating involuntary treatment. Dismissing or reducing the charges is typical if the defendant meets the treatment requirements.

In New York, there was a significant reduction in the rate of re-arrest (33%), readmission (45%), and return to prison (87%) compared to inmates who did not participate in the drug court program.

In California, federal costs per drug-related prisoner average $11,000 per year. But when a drug-related offender fulfills a California drug court order, the price per inmate drops to just $3,000 per year. Researchers are observing similar results in many other states.

About 137,000 people are in state prisons or jails in the United States on any given day for drug possession, often for possession of small amounts of illegal drugs.

More than half of people in state prisons and two-thirds of those awaiting prison sentencing have a problem with drug use or meet the criteria for addiction. Additionally, people with addiction face prison terms, but access to evidence-based treatment is minimal.

With greater oversight and the threat of imprisonment, offenders can receive treatment for about twice as long (e.g., from 30 days to 60 days treatment) as voluntary community drug programs. On the other hand, the more court-ordered treatments, the fewer beds are available to the general population. Unfortunately, those not integrated into the legal system will have fewer treatment options.

FUNDING: More incentives are needed for providers to open complementary treatment plans. There are not enough resources to provide addiction treatment. In a 2010 study, there were 46 million addicts in the USA.

"The addiction crisis is deadlier than ever before. Overdoses are the #1 cause of accidental death in our country. According to the CDC, there were over 107,000 fatal overdoses in the US in 2021. That's the highest number of overdose deaths ever recorded in a single year." (Shatterproof)[89]

Effective behavioral and substance addiction treatment is difficult to access and rarely covered by insurance. Only 1 in 10 people who need treatment get treatment, let alone get high-quality care based on scientific evidence.

ABSTINENCE vs. HARM REDUCTION: There is an ongoing disagreement between abstinence-based recovery and harm reduction as a therapeutic philosophy. Abstinence-based recovery is no use. In contrast, harm reduction strategies aim to decrease substance use gradually. This approach may include the use of controlled substances, such as replacing heroin with methadone, a less potent opiate, to manage withdrawal symptoms and reduce the risk associated with more dangerous drugs.

Most addiction counselors believe that users who cross the line and engage in uncontrolled drug use or compulsions can easily refuse the first drink, shot, or gambling but cannot refuse the second. These

---

[89] Shatterproof (n.a.) (2024) Retrieved from https://www.shatterproof.org/learn/addiction-basics/addiction-in-america

experts believe that abstinence is essential for recovery because the very definition of addiction is the loss of self-control.

Haight Ashbury, Free Clinics studies, showed, "When a client slipped (e.g., had a drink, took one hit, or smoked one cigarette), it turned into a full relapse in 95% of the cases."[90]

On the other hand, harm reduction is the willingness to work towards gradual change rather than demanding a complete behavior change. Mitigation includes:

- Drug Replacement Therapy, such as methadone or Suboxone maintenance therapy instead of heroin use or methylphenidate maintenance therapy instead of cocaine use.
- Needle Exchange: safe injection sites and distribution of naloxone to opiate addicts.
- Designated Drivers: non-drinking or non-drug drivers, wet hostels or sobering stations.
- Substitution: replacing more harmful drugs with less harmful drugs, such as cannabis, instead of heroin.
- Drug Quality Testing: testing illegal drugs before use, preventing the use of disguised substances such as fentanyl.
- Drinking or Drugging Age Requirements: lowering age requirements for alcohol and drugs to give young people more time to mature through experience.
- Decriminalization of Drugs through legalization and legislation.
- Use of Controlled Substances through behavior modification

Long-term follow-up clearly shows that controlled drinking doesn't work. Most treatment centers effectively adopt an abstinence-based philosophy incorporating various harm reduction techniques.

Chemical addiction is the number one health and social problem worldwide despite being one of the most treatable problems. Successful participation in treatment programs results in more extended abstinence,

---

[90] Ibid, Inaba, Craig, 442

healthier minds and bodies, social improvements, and psychological benefits for participants.

The Decriminalization of Drug Offenses

David Sheff, in his 2013 publication "Clean: Overcoming Addiction and Ending America's Greatest Tragedy," presents the argument that addiction ought to be approached and managed as a health concern rather than being perceived as a moral shortcoming or a form of criminal behavior. This viewpoint is pivotal for a variety of reasons. Initially, it removes the stigma associated with addiction, encouraging people to pursue assistance free from embarrassment or apprehension. Furthermore, it advocates for using treatments based on scientific evidence instead of resorting to punitive actions. Sheff underscores the significance of recognizing addiction as a persistent illness that necessitates comprehensive and sustained treatment strategies.[91]

A critical element of Sheff's discourse is the influence of societal perceptions and public policies in tackling addiction. He scrutinizes the war on drugs and the criminal justice system's treatment of addiction, pointing out that these strategies have frequently aggravated the issue instead of mitigating it. Sheff advocates for a transition to a more empathetic and health-oriented approach and emphasizes the necessity for widespread systemic reform.

A Biblical Step 1: We admitted we were powerless over alcohol [addiction]; our lives were beyond our control. Step one tells us we must acknowledge our inability to heal ourselves and our need for a Savior.[92]

---

[91] Sheff, D. (2013). Clean: Overcoming addiction and ending America's greatest tragedy. Houghton Mifflin Harcourt.

[92] Jennings, T. Retrieved from file:///Users/pierresamaan/Documents/My Files/SubstDis/JENNINGS/Biblical Approach to Addictions.html

The Bibles Says...

Jesus heard what they said and replied, "Those who believe they are healthy don't go to the doctor; only the sick do. I cannot help those who believe they are already right with God, but only those who know they are sick with sin." (Mark 2:17 REM)

CHAPTER 11

UNMASKING RECOVERY — ACCEPTING FOR DENIAL ON THE ROAD TO RECOVERY!

Proper recovery from substance and behavioral addictions begins with an individual's recognition that they have hit rock bottom. Addiction is the only disease that requires self-diagnosis to be effective in treatment, even if others perceive it as addiction.

Previously, we ended with the Biblical Step 1; we admitted that we were powerless over alcohol [addiction]; our lives were beyond our control. Step one tells us we must acknowledge our inability to heal ourselves and our need for a Savior.[93]

What Is Denial?

Denial, within the context of AA 12-step programs, is a concept that holds immense importance. It is not only recognized as a common defense mechanism but also as a powerful obstacle to overcome in the journey toward addiction recovery. Consequently, denial plays a significant role in shaping these programs' first, fourth, fifth, eighth, and tenth steps. Through confronting and dismantling denial, individuals can pave the way for a transformative healing process.

---

[93] Jennings, T. Retrieved from file:///Users/pierresamaan/Documents/My Files/SubstDis/JENNINGS/Biblical Approach to Addictions.html

At its core, denial manifests as the steadfast refusal to acknowledge the detrimental effects brought about by addiction or the abuse of addictive substances and behaviors. It is a state of mind that seeks to negate or contradict the truth—consciously or unconsciously. In the eyes of others, denial may often be perceived as a refusal to face reality or a reluctance to take responsibility for one's actions. However, it goes beyond mere defiance and can be seen as a rebellious act that challenges both human authority and the divine laws established by God.

Understanding denial within the realms of addiction and recovery necessitates a holistic approach that draws from various sources of wisdom and insight. Numerous references in the Bible and Christian teachings shed light on the significance of acknowledging and rectifying denial.

Denial Is Fear-based

Despite the overwhelming evidence, claiming that something isn't true is a form of self-defense, self-protection, and selfishness based on a belief in fear.

Fear and anxiety can be natural, like when a doctor declares you have a terminal illness. People who show symptoms of a severe disease sometimes deny or ignore those symptoms because the thought of a serious health problem causes fear, discomfort, and anxiety.

However, in substance and behavioral abuse or dependency, denial defense mechanisms are based on self-protection, with a strong bias towards selfishness. They don't want to admit they have an addiction disorder and don't want to give up the pleasure of getting drunk and running away, even if it means they are likely to hurt themselves or others.

Believing lies negatively expands imaginations, expanding the brain's fear circuitry. Fear is part of the limbic system or what I often call the "basement" of the brain. Fear paralyzes part of the prefrontal cortex, the "upper room" of the brain.

Imagine an individual who is terrified of exams or public speaking. When confronted with these situations, they become paralyzed by fear, unable to articulate their thoughts or speak coherently. They require assistance to process their thoughts clearly or express themselves fluently. Similarly, individuals in denial experience a comparable paralysis. Anxiety rooted in fear hinders their ability to think clearly, leading to impaired judgment and difficulty in solving problems.

Despite evidence to the contrary, the poor choices of believing lies strengthen the circuits of the limbic system. In doing so, we are breaking God's laws, repeatedly disenfranchising ourselves, and severely limiting our freedom. God is not doing it to us; we are doing it ourselves.

Fear-based denial in addiction recovery is a phenomenon where individuals refuse to acknowledge or accept their addiction or the severity of their addiction due to fear. This fear can stem from various sources, including the fear of change, fear of facing the consequences of one's actions, fear of losing the coping mechanism that the addiction provides, or fear of stigma and judgment. Understanding this concept is crucial in addiction recovery counseling, focusing on providing comprehensive and compassionate care.

Primary among the critical aspects of fear-based denial is *Fear of Change*. Many individuals in addiction may fear the unknown elements of life without their substance or behavior of choice. This fear can lead to denial as a defense mechanism (Simpson & Miller, 2002).[94]

More often than not, the *Fear of Confronting Past Traumas* comes into play. Addictions often serve as coping mechanisms for underlying issues such as trauma or mental health disorders. Acknowledging the addiction might mean confronting these painful experiences (Maté, 2008).[95]

The *Fear of Stigma* surrounding addiction can lead individuals to deny their problem to avoid judgment or "ostracization" (Luoma et al., 2007).[96]

---

[94] Simpson, D. D., & Miller, M. (2002). Confronting the paradoxes of motivation to change: The many faces of denial in addictions treatment. *Addiction, 97*(9), 1207-1213.

[95] Maté, G. (2008). In the realm of hungry ghosts: Close encounters with addiction. North Atlantic Books.

[96] Luoma, J. B., Twohig, M. P., Waltz, T., Hayes, S. C., Roget, N., Padilla, M., & Fisher, G. (2007). An investigation of stigma in individuals receiving treatment for substance abuse. *Addictive Behaviors, 32*(7), 1331-1346.

For some, their *Fear of Losing a Coping Mechanism* can be unthinkable. For the addict, a coping mechanism, such as a substance or addictive behavior, is a way to manage stress, emotions, or mental health issues. Losing this can be frightening, reinforcing denial (Khantzian, 1997).[97]

There are many reasons for fear-based denial, including *Fear of Responsibility and Consequences.* Acknowledging an addiction might mean facing the consequences of one's actions, which can be daunting (Marlatt & Donovan, 2005).[98]

Cognitive Behavioral Theory (CBT) suggests that denial is a cognitive distortion where individuals rationalize or justify their addictive behavior (Beck, 1993).[99]

Psychodynamic Theory views denial as a defense mechanism to protect the ego from anxiety and internal conflict (Freud, 1923).[100]

Denial, as understood from the perspective of Learning Theory, is a psychological defense mechanism where an individual refuses to acknowledge the reality of a stressful or anxiety-inducing situation. This concept is more commonly discussed in psychoanalytic theory, but it can also be examined from a Learning Theory standpoint.

In the context of Learning Theory, denial can be understood as a learned behavior where an individual refuses to acknowledge the reality of a stressful or anxiety-inducing situation. This perspective suggests that individuals may learn to deny reality as a coping mechanism in response to adverse or traumatic situations. The behavior of denial is reinforced when it successfully reduces anxiety or discomfort, even though it may not be an adaptive or healthy long-term strategy (Skinner 1953).[101]

Albert Bandura's Social Learning Theory provides insight into

[97] Khantzian, E. J. (1997). The self-medication hypothesis of substance use disorders: A reconsideration and recent applications. *Harvard Review of Psychiatry, 4*(5), 231-244.

[98] Marlatt, G. A., & Donovan, D. M. (Eds.). (2005). Relapse prevention: Maintenance strategies in the treatment of addictive behaviors. Guilford Press.

[99] Beck, A. T. (1993). Cognitive therapy: Nature and relation to behavior therapy. *Behavior Therapy, 24*(4), 621-624.

[100] Freud, S. (1923). The ego and the id. *SE*, 19: 1-66.

[101] Skinner, B. F. (1953). *Science and Human Behavior*. Macmillan.

denial. This theory emphasizes learning through observation and imitation. If an individual observes others successfully employing denial to avoid discomfort, they may imitate this behavior, learning to use denial themselves (Bandura 1977).[102]

In considering the subject matter, it is valuable to acknowledge the profound insights that can be gleaned from the Bible and Christian doctrinal teachings, particularly concerning fear-based denial. This psychological defense mechanism is characterized by an individual's refusal to acknowledge or confront a distressing reality driven by underlying fear. Such a response is not just a psychological construct but also finds resonance within the scriptural context. The Bible provides a rich tapestry of teachings and narratives that delve into the nature of fear, the pursuit of truth, and the dynamics of denial in diverse scenarios.

Biblical insights emphasize fear-based denial's spiritual and moral dimensions, offering a deeper understanding of this behavior. The scriptures frequently address the human tendency to evade truth due to fear, underscoring the spiritual implications of such avoidance. They encourage a confrontation with truth as a pathway to liberation and spiritual growth in alignment with Christian principles. This perspective enhances the mental and emotional understanding of fear-based denial and enriches it with spiritual and ethical considerations, providing a more holistic approach to addressing this phenomenon.

Integrating biblical wisdom with mental and emotional concepts like fear-based denial enables a more comprehensive exploration of human behavior, blending spiritual, mental, and emotional dimensions. This approach aligns with the Christian belief in the interconnection of spirit, soul, and body, advocating for a balanced and truth-oriented life.

This perspective is corroborated by various sources, including psychological studies on defense mechanisms and theological analyses of biblical teachings related to fear and truth. For instance, the works

---

[102] Bandura, A. (1977). "Social Learning Theory". Englewood Cliffs, NJ: Prentice Hall.

of renowned psychiatrists and psychologists such as Sigmund Freud and Anna Freud on defense mechanisms provide a foundational understanding of fear-based denial. Simultaneously, theological discussions, such as those in commentaries on biblical passages dealing with fear and truth, offer spiritual insights into this behavior.

The merging of biblical teachings with mental and emotional principles offers a nuanced and enriched understanding of fear-based denial, highlighting its multifaceted nature and encouraging a comprehensive approach to addressing it.

The Holy Scriptures frequently discuss managing fear and its effects. A notable verse, 2 Timothy 1:7, declares, *"For God has not given us a spirit of fear, but of power and of love and of a sound mind."* This scripture highlights that a life of fear is incompatible with Christian principles founded on power, love, and mental clarity.

The Bible consistently underscores the necessity of confronting the truth in denial and truth. As Jesus articulates in John 8:32, *"And you will know the truth, and the truth will set you free,"* it is evident that embracing and accepting truth is essential for spiritual liberation. In contrast, denial is portrayed as an obstacle to achieving this freedom.

Biblical narratives provide several examples of fear-based denial. The incident of Peter denying Jesus (Matthew 26:69-75) is a prime example. Here, Peter, overwhelmed by fear for his safety, disowns Jesus, a decision he later profoundly regrets. This episode underscores the harmful nature of fear-driven denial and the significance of countering fear with faith.

The Bible also offers counsel on surmounting fear through reliance on God. As expressed in Psalm 34:4 (NIV), *"I sought the Lord, and he answered me; he delivered me from all my fears,"* seeking God is suggested as an effective means of conquering fear. This reliance on divine strength, rather than human capability, is a central motif in biblical doctrine.

Furthermore, the New Testament highlights the importance of communal support among Christians in facing fear and denial. Galatians 6:2 urges, *"Bear one another's burdens, and so fulfill the law of*

Christ" (NIV), signifying the Christian duty to support and guide one another in times of fear and denial.

Treatment Implications

Compassionate Confrontation is a counseling approach that gently challenges the client's denial while showing understanding and empathy. This technique is particularly effective when clients resist acknowledging problematic behaviors or thought patterns. In cases of addiction, this approach can help clients recognize their harmful patterns while reassuring them of God's love and forgiveness. The essence of Compassionate Confrontation lies in its balanced approach — it is neither overly aggressive nor excessively permissive. This method aligns well with the principles of Christian counseling, which emphasize love, understanding, and the pursuit of truth (Miller & Rollnick, 2002).[103]

Continuing from the concept of Motivational Interviewing (MI), a client-centered counseling style for eliciting behavior change by helping clients explore and resolve ambivalence, it's essential to delve deeper into its methodologies and applications, especially in Clinical Christian Counseling (Miller & Rollnick, 2002).[104]

MI is grounded in a compassionate and empathic approach. It involves understanding the client's perspective and feelings without judgment. This aligns with the Christian values of compassion and understanding as highlighted in scriptures like Colossians 3:12, which encourages believers to clothe themselves with compassion, kindness, humility, gentleness, and patience.

MI focuses on helping clients perceive the discrepancies between their current behavior and their broader life values and goals. This method resonates with the Christian principle of self-reflection and aligning one's actions with one's faith and values.

Instead of confronting or opposing resistance, MI advises practitioners to accept and understand resistance as a natural part of

---

[103] Miller, W. R., & Rollnick, S. (2002). Motivational interviewing: Preparing people for change. Guilford Press.
[104] Ibid.

the change process. This is similar to the Christian ethos of patience and understanding in facing challenges, as advised in James 1:19-20.

MI places significant emphasis on the belief that individuals have the power to change. It parallels the Christian belief in personal agency and the transformative power of faith (Philippians 4:13).

Motivational Interviewing can be particularly effective in dealing with addictions, a common area of focus in Christian counseling. It helps clients find the motivation to change by connecting their desire to overcome addiction with their spiritual goals.

Cognitive-behavioral therapy (CBT) is a form of counseling that focuses on the relationship between thoughts, feelings, and behaviors. It is rooted in the fundamental principle that our thoughts and perceptions influence our emotional and behavioral responses. In the context of addiction treatment, CBT aims to help clients recognize and modify maladaptive thought patterns and behaviors that contribute to substance abuse (Beck, 1993).[105]

Integrating these biblical insights can be helpful from a Christian counseling perspective. Encouraging clients to confront their fears, lean on their faith, and seek support from their community can be part of a holistic approach to dealing with fear-based denial. While the Bible provides guidance, it's important to remember that fear-based denial can also have complex psychological roots. Counseling may sometimes be necessary to address underlying issues.

The biblical perspective on fear-based denial involves recognizing the detrimental effects of fear, the importance of facing the truth, relying on faith in God to overcome fear, and seeking support from the Christian community. This perspective can be integrated into Christian counseling practices to help individuals confront and overcome their fears in a spiritually and emotionally healthy manner.

---

[105] Beck, A. T. (1993). Cognitive therapy: Nature and relation to behavior therapy. *Behavior Therapy, 24*(4), 621-624.

Eliciting Love as a Way-Out of Fear-Based Denial

Of course, those who care about healing the addictive client cannot force change by violating God-given free will. Let's learn from the biblical description of the character of God, who is truth, love, and freedom. Evidence presented in love gives freedom to agree or disagree. Change that is grown out of fear will not elicit love but rebellion.

God's truths are weapons against denial. *"For the word of God is the living and active revelation of the truth about God, his methods and principles, and the real basis of life in the universe. It is sharper than any two-edged sword: it penetrates the deepest recesses of the mind and separates thoughts and feelings, habits and motives; it also diagnoses the true intentions, attitudes, and principles of the heart. Nothing in all creation is hidden from God's sight, as he knows the true condition of our minds. Everything is open and clearly seen by him who will one day examine and accurately diagnose us all."* (Hebrews 4:12-13 REM)

There is something special about God's truths. His Truths are so revealing to our hearts and minds they act like a burning fire to the soul. When tilling the soil, seeds take root and thrive—preparing the earth through a labor of love for seeds to take root.

What method or gateway does God use to bring about this healing in us individually? What is the way to your heart and my heart? Your sound judgment is a combination of reason and conscience (Isaiah 1:18). This is how the truth enters our thoughts, and then we reflect and decide whether or not to form our beliefs. Our beliefs shape our character, values, attitudes, brain circuits, and how we process and understand new facts and truths.

Psychiatrist T. R. Jennings, MD, says, "The righteous will be transformed by this life-giving glory — as Moses was after 40 days with God. Moses came down off the mountain, and his face was radiating this fiery glory (Ex 34:29-35). But did Moses have 3rd-degree burns? No, the fire was not harmful. But what about the children of Israel? When they saw Moses, what did they do? They begged him to put a veil over his face because this light caused them anguish and suffering. But what kind of suffering? Suffering of mind. Why? Because their consciences were guilty, because they didn't value God's methods and principles, because they preferred lies and selfishness; the light of heavenly love and truth caused them to suffer." (Jennings 2008)[106]

In scriptural texts, the term 'brimstone' or 'sulfur' is derived from the Greek words "thion" or "thios," which signify divinity or the sacred nature of the Godhead (Kittel & Friedrich, 1965-1976). This linguistic root extends into the English word "theology," which denotes the study of divine and sacred matters. Consequently, the biblical expression "fire and brimstone" might be more accurately rendered as "divine incense" or "holy fire," emphasizing a celestial rather than destructive quality.[107]

Once again, we come back to the understanding that the fire of God's presence is what is represented and not burning brimstone! Could these be the same fiery stones Lucifer walked between before his fall, as described in Ezekiel 28:14? Could it be the fire Elijah rode in as the chariot of fire carried him to heaven (2 Kings 2:11)?

We find another example in Leviticus 10:1-5, where Aaron's entitled sons Nabad and Abide, without permission, in rebellion, brought fire before God. They were destroyed not by an explosive fire but by the fire of God's truth, shocking their minds and bodies to death. Because of their desire to resist authority, the fire of truth and exposure from God consumed them — sudden death by short-circuiting intensity of the brain's fear circuitry.

We know it was not combustion because their bodies were carried out, still in their tunics — no combustibly burnt clothing or bodies. The presence of God will either cleanse the hearts and minds of those who "know" Him through His son, Jesus Christ, or they become consumed by the fiery flashing of His truth.

That fire is an illuminating fire of truth & love (representative of Jesus Christ), completely overwhelming the hearts and minds of those without sorrow and unchangeable — unrepentant.

What will those who have hardened their hearts with lies and

---

[106] Jennings, T. (2008) "The Question of Punishment" —Part 3. Retrieved from https://comeandreason.com/the-question-of-punishment-part-iii/
[107] Kittel, G., & Friedrich, G. (Eds.). (1964-1976). Theological Dictionary of the New Testament. Eerdmans.

selfishness (fear-based denial) do when Christ appears, confronting them with undiluted, infinite truth and love?

Emotional trauma can indeed precipitate a genuine cardiac condition akin to a broken heart. This phenomenon was substantiated through research at Johns Hopkins University School of Medicine, revealing that abrupt emotional stress can lead to a reversible form of heart failure. Dr. Ilan Wittstein, a cardiologist at Hopkins and principal investigator of this study, which has been featured in the New England Journal of Medicine, expounded on this. In an analysis of 19 instances of what's termed "broken heart syndrome" from 1999 to 2003, a correlation was established between intense emotional distress and cardiac dysfunction in individuals who were previously heart-healthy (Keyvan 2005).[108]

The study underscored that the catalyst for such cardiac distress is often a profoundly distressing event, not a mere disappointment. Instances like relationship terminations, the demise of a loved one, or even the shock from a surprise event can trigger cardiac incidents in individuals with no prior heart disease, suggesting their generally sound health. Interestingly, these cases often necessitate only brief medical intervention, as the heart tends to recuperate naturally.

Dr. Wittstein, in his interactions with Denise Grady of the New York Times and Rob Stein of the Washington Post, emphasized the tangible impact of emotional stress on the heart. He highlighted the potential lethality of a broken heart, attributing it to a unique mechanism of heart attack. Medical practitioners often misidentify these heart attacks, mistaking them for those caused by poor physical health rather than emotional trauma.

The underlying cause is an abundance of stress hormones, leading to severe weakening of the heart muscle. This condition is medically termed stress cardiomyopathy, though it is more colloquially known

---

[108] Keyvan, N. (2005) Emotional shock really can lead to a broken heart. A study at Johns Hopkins University School of Medicine has demonstrated that sudden emotional stress can result in reversible heart failure. https://www.jhunewsletter.com/article/2005/03/sudden-shock-can-lead-to-heart-attack-81296

as "broken heart" syndrome. In this state, the heart's ability to pump blood effectively is temporarily compromised.

The concept of excited delirium syndrome (ExDS) often emerges in discussions about fear-based denial, particularly in the context of extreme stress or mental health crises. ExDS is a controversial term primarily used in emergency medicine and law enforcement. It describes a state where an individual exhibits highly agitated and aggressive behavior, often combined with hallucinations, paranoia, and a seeming imperviousness to pain.

The intensification of fear-based denial can be seen as a psychological mechanism where an individual, facing extreme stress or a traumatic event, resorts to denying reality as a way of coping. This denial can manifest in various forms, from ignoring the situation to adopting counterproductive or dangerous behaviors.

In the context of ExDS, this denial can exacerbate the situation, as the affected individual is not only experiencing intense physiological and psychological symptoms but also potentially denying the severity of their condition or the reality of their circumstances. This can lead to a dangerous escalation of the situation, posing risks to the individual and those around them.

In the last ten years, the concept of *excited delirium syndrome* (ExDS) has been a subject of ongoing debate, particularly in cases involving the death of highly agitated individuals while in police custody, restrained, or subdued with electrical devices. During post-mortem examinations, forensic pathologists often struggle to pinpoint an apparent anatomical reason for death. However, the intoxication from psychostimulants is regularly mentioned as a contributing factor. ExDS is typically characterized by a range of symptoms, including erratic and aggressive behavior, loud shouting, paranoia, panic attacks, violence, unexpected physical strength, and elevated body temperature (Mash 2016).[109]

These symptoms closely mirror those observed in acute exhaustive

---

[109] Mash, D. (2016) Excited Delirium and Sudden Death: A Syndromal Disorder at the Extreme End of the Neuropsychiatric Continuum. Front Physiol. 2016; 7: 435. Published online 2016 Oct 13. doi: 10.3389/fphys.2016.00435 https://www.ncbi.nlm. nih.gov/pmc/articles/PMC5061757/

mania and sudden death scenarios, especially in individuals abusing psychostimulants or in other sudden death cases. Post-mortem neurochemical examinations of brain tissues in such instances have revealed significant findings. There is a noted disruption in the regulation of the dopamine transporter system, coupled with increased levels of heat shock protein 70 (hsp70), indicative of hyperthermia.

The sudden demise of individuals suffering from ExDS is increasingly being understood in biological terms. Elevated levels of dopamine in the brain can trigger extreme manic and hysterical states. If these states are not controlled, they can lead to a breakdown in autonomic regulation, eventually progressing to a catastrophic failure of the cardiorespiratory system. This insight into the biophysical mechanisms underlying ExDS highlights the complex interplay of neurochemical imbalances and physiological responses that can culminate in fatal outcomes.

Revelation 6:15-16 tells us that all the kings, princes, generals, wealthy, mighty, enslaved people, and free men of the earth hid in caves and among the rocks of the mountains. They called for the mountains and rocks to "fall upon us" and "hide us" from the face of God and the wrath of the Lamb who sits on his throne! — Wrath can also mean recognizing God's cleansing fire of truth & love.

You can never escape the truth; you can only delay the day you deal with it.

On the path to successful addiction treatment, the immediate solution to fear-based denial is to remove fear, selfishness, and sin (wrongdoing) from the heart and soul. Recognizing truth evidenced by enduring change only happens when Jesus Christ is centered.

Most often, the evidence of a successful prevalence of the gospel of Jesus Christ in treatment and recovery programs will be the long-lasting sobriety rate of two years or more after treatment among those undergoing spiritual/biblical recovery versus others.

Thwarting Denial

When people open their hearts to God, their interest in change and reconciliation increases. As the substance or behaviorally addicted client gains knowledge of God in his biblical recovery, he develops a strong desire to emulate the love of God demonstrated throughout the earthly life of the Son of God, Jesus Christ.

At the same time, the addict becomes closer in love with God and with each other. A Christ-centered, Bible-based, scientifically supported recovery helps clients grow in knowledge and spiritual awareness, manifesting mature spiritual fruition in unity and patience. *"It was he [Jesus] who selected some as his ambassadors, some to be spokespersons, some to be preachers of the healing message, some to care for and minister to his children, and some to educate and instruct— all in order to heal God's people, enabling them to help each other — so that the body of believers may grow in number and strength until we all reach true unity of heart, methods, motives and principles in harmony with the knowledge of God as revealed in Jesus, and become mature, developing Christlike character."* (Ephesians 4: 11-13 REM; emphasis pjs).

Coming out of denial to begin recovery begins with accepting your Savior, Jesus, making Him the center of all life, and following only His ways and principles in your relationships with others—God's law of love.

A Biblical Step 2...

☑ We must know the truth about God — He is in the saving business, not the condemning business, and He can heal us. (Matthew 11:28-30; Revelations 3:20)

We decided to turn our will and lives to God's care as we understood Him.

The Bible Says...

"The devil tempts us through our emotions, so don't give him any opportunity to confuse you or lead you astray. The person who has been stealing [or, in addictions] has been practicing the methods of selfishness, and if they desire to get well, they must have selfishness replaced by love. When selfishness is replaced with love, they will stop stealing, and instead get a job in order to be able to give to others in need." (Ephesians 4:27-28 REM) (Brackets added)

CHAPTER 12

UNMASKING RECOVERY —
THE FOUR PHASES OF RECOVERY!

Four Phases of Recovery

In recovery from a drug or behavioral addiction, clients undergo four stages: detoxification, initial abstinence, long-term abstinence/sobriety, and continuous recovery. A crucial phase is Detoxification because without the body metabolizing the toxic drug out of the body, there can be no benefit from treatment.

Phase 1: Detoxification

Detoxification is the first step in addiction treatment. If the client is still consuming, the drug must be removed or detoxified from the body. Whether the client depends on the substance or behavior, the body's chemistry or biochemistry is out of balance.

In the initial detoxification phase, unpleasant physical and psychological symptoms occur after stopping or reducing the substance, so-called withdrawal symptoms. The characteristics of withdrawal syndrome depend on which drug is being discontinued. Symptoms include anxiety, fatigue, sweating, vomiting, depression, seizures, and hallucinations.

Mental and emotional withdrawal encompasses the psychological consequences of stopping the use of an addictive substance. It can also occur when someone gives up a habit such as compulsive shopping, gambling, or viewing pornography.

According to the Substance Abuse and Mental Health Administration (SAMHSA), there are three types of withdrawal: acute withdrawal, protracted (long-term) withdrawal, and post-acute-protracted syndrome.

The first type of detoxification, acute withdrawal, consists mainly of physical withdrawal symptoms that last from a few days to two weeks. Acute withdrawal symptoms are immediate or initial withdrawal symptoms that occur when the use of addictive substances, including alcohol, is abruptly stopped or rapidly reduced.

Delirium Tremens (DT) is the most severe type of withdrawal syndrome. Signs and symptoms include extreme confusion, excitement, and agitation — severely elevated mood.

A long-term or protracted withdrawal syndrome can develop, in which symptoms persist for months to years after the substance is stopped. Benzodiazepines, opioids, alcohol, and all other drugs, such as psychedelics, can lead to long-term withdrawal or similar effects, and symptoms can persist for years after use has stopped.

Post-acute-protracted syndrome (PAWS) is most commonly called **permanent withdrawal syndrome**. PAWS may also be called post-withdrawal syndrome, prolonged withdrawal syndrome, or protracted (prolonged) withdrawal syndrome.

The most common symptoms of PAWS include difficulties with cognitive tasks such as learning, problem-solving, and memory—irritability; feelings of fear and panic; and depression.

Withdrawal Risk Factors During Detox

Access for the following associated with increased patient risk for complicated withdrawal or complications of withdrawal:[110]

---

[110] Retrieved from http://eguideline.guidelinecentral.com/i/1254278-alcohol-withdrawal-management/5?

- History of alcohol or drug withdrawal, delirium, or seizures.
- Numerous prior withdrawal episodes in the patient's lifetime
- Comorbid medical or surgical illness (especially traumatic brain injury)
- Increased age (>65); moderate to severe active and potentially destabilizing medical problems, including unstable chronic condition. Suspected head injury. Unable to take oral medications.
- Long duration of heavy and regular alcohol or drug consumption
- Seizure(s) during the current withdrawal episode; (>8 standard drinks per day)
- Marked autonomic hyperactivity on presentation
- Physiological dependence on GABAergic agents such as benzodiazepines or barbiturates—What are GABAergic agents? GABA stands for gamma-aminobutyric acid, which is a neurotransmitter. GABAergic agents are medicines that affect the level of GABA in the brain.
- Concomitant use of other addictive substances (Withdrawing from other substances)
- Positive blood alcohol concentration in the presence of signs and symptoms of withdrawal
- Signs or symptoms of a co-occurring psychiatric disorder are active and reflect moderate severity.
- Risk of harm: Commitment is low, and cooperation and reliability are questionable. Imminent risk of injury—not cooperative or reliable. Significant threat of imminent relapse.

Drug Detection

Each drug works differently depending on the type of drug test used. The two most common point-of-use drug testing methods are saliva and urine. Other factors influencing drug detection periods include a person's weight, tolerance for the drug, method of drug use, activity, diet, metabolic rate, age, and urine PH.

Understanding the detection times of different substances and differences in testing methods is critical to choosing the type of test for your situation. The saliva test is a late indicator of drug use, while urinalysis can expand the detection window. The point-of-collection test is a preliminary drug screening method, and a laboratory must confirm any initial positive result.

When Are Prescriptions Necessary For Detox?

Medical care during treatment during detoxification may require a medically controlled inpatient facility. Medically or chemically assisted detoxification aims to minimize withdrawal symptoms that can cause life-threatening effects or immediate relapse.

Assessing the severity of drug toxicity is vital in determining the need for medical detoxification. The degree of addiction, the likelihood of severe withdrawal symptoms, the presence of other medical or psychological problems, the patient's response to recommended treatments, the possibility of relapse, and the environment for recovery must all be determined.

Various drugs will alleviate withdrawal symptoms during detoxification and minimize initial drug cravings. Also, using some of the same medications is helpful during the initial abstinence, long-term abstinence, and recovery phases. Below is a list of common prescriptions used during detox:[111]

- **Clonidine** (catapres) dampens the withdrawal symptoms of opioids, alcohol, and nicotine addiction.
- **Phenobarbital** or chlordiazepoxide (Librium) prevents withdrawal seizures and other symptoms associated with alcohol and sedative-hypnotic dependence.
- **Methadone**, a long-acting opioid, is one of four feral-approved medications for opioid addiction treatment (for detoxification

---

[111] Inaba, Craig, (2014) "Uppers, Downers, All Arounders," 8th Edition, p. 456, CNS Publications, Ashland, OR

and maintenance). The other three are buprenorphine, LAAM, and naltrexone.

- **Buprenorphine** (Subutex and Suboxone) can be used for short-term opioid detoxification or long-term maintenance.
- **Naltrexone** (ReVia), or in its injectable form, Vivitrol blocks the effects of opioids. It is also used during alcohol detoxification. The drug blocks the response to heroin if the addict slips while in treatment; it also blocks cravings for alcohol and opiates, making it useful in relapse prevention. Some clinicians also use it to block cravings in stimulant abuse, gambling, and other addictive disorders.
- **Psychiatric medications**, including antipsychotics such as haloperidol (Haldol), antidepressants such as desipramine and imipramine (Tofranil), and selective serotonin reuptake inhibitor (SSRI) Antidepressants such as Sertraline (Zoloft) and fluoxetine (Prozac), are used in the initial detoxification of cocaine, amphetamine, and other stimulant addictions.
- **Anticonvulsant medications** such as topiramate (Topamax) and gabapentin (Neurontin) control cravings to prevent alcohol or stimulant abuse relapse.

Social or non-medical supervised programs require clients to undergo either medical detoxification or be 72 hours clean and sober on their own before treatment and admission.

Treatment includes supportive care and medications to address symptoms and prevent complications.

A Biblical Step 3

☑ We open our hearts to God and let His power transform and heal us from within. We made a searching and fearless moral inventory of ourselves.

The Bible Says...

"Examine me, O God, and know the deepest recesses of my heart, test me and identify every troublesome thought. Determine if there is any unhealthy way in me, and lead me back to everlasting life." (Psalm 139:23-24 REM)

Phase 2: Initial Abstinence

Earlier, we talked about the first stage of recovery treatment, detoxification. The remaining three improve knowledge, understanding, and insight skills. After an agonizing detoxification period, initial abstinence, prolonged abstinence/sobriety, and continued recovery follow.

Once the addict is clear of toxic substances, a period of rehabilitation begins called initial abstinence or early abstinence. We can define abstinence as refraining from something or not doing or having something that is wanted or enjoyable.

After physical and mental detoxification, Substance Use Disorder (SUD)'s initial abstinence stage consists of mindlessness and emotional flooding. An incomplete detox increases the fear and vulnerability that arises from memories and trauma, leading to emotional flooding.

According to the Gottman Institute, flooding is "a sensation of feeling psychologically and physically overwhelmed during conflict, making it virtually impossible to have a productive, problem-solving discussion."[112]

In the early stages of recovery, it can be overwhelming when the body senses danger. For many, just a difficult conversation, harsh feedback, or a straightforward discussion strains our bodies, making it easy to feel overwhelmed, attacked, and confused.

During emotional flooding, powerful thoughts and emotions trigger an influx of physiological sensations and a surge in the stress hormones adrenaline and cortisol — defense mode. Threatening

---

[112] Retrieved from https://www.gottman.com/blog/brene-browns-atlas-of-the-heart-defensiveness-and-flooding/

perceptions leading to self-protection can make it challenging to access self-restraint.

Early abstinence may vary in severity due to incomplete detoxification. It takes time for your body chemistry to balance. Continued sobriety during the initial abstinence is best encouraged by addressing the addict's constant cravings and aspects of the addict's life that may pose a risk of relapse.

Medical approaches used during a detox may need to continue to curb and reverse the pleasurable effects of drugs, reduce drug cravings, and encourage addicts to stay clean, but it is not for everyone.

Anti-craving medications, such as those used during the detox phase, can also be continued during the more traditional approach, the early abstinence phase. Voluntary isolation from environmental triggers and cues (bars, fellow users, drug paraphernalia, etc.), counseling, and 12-step meetings are ineffective in controlling episodic drug cravings.

The persistent change in brain chemistry and circuitry brought about by drug or behavioral addiction creates a vulnerability to relapse long after the drug or behavior has ceased. In other words, the brain's reward system has morphed into an "anti-reward" system.[113]

What is an anti-reward system? In response to the overuse of the brain's reward system, the addict's brain's anti-reward system becomes overactive, causing a severe dysphoric phase (mood, dissatisfaction, irritability) when the direct effects of the drug wear off. As a result, persistent changes in motivation bring an associated tendency to relapse into addiction; "I need to feel good again!"

Substance use and abuse (or addictive behavior changing brain chemistry) create persistent cravings resulting from the breakdown of neurotransmitters in the brain. The breakdown is known as an "endogenous" craving.

Endogenous craving activates the brain's hippocampus, which is essential for memory, and helps reinforce the reward-seeking behaviors that give us a powerful desire — craving. Pre-existing opioid receptors in the brain turn on and create an inner craving from the memories. Frequent and intense addictive experiences produce stronger cravings.

---

[113] Retrieved from https://pubmed.ncbi.nlm.nih.gov/18154498/

Taking alcohol as an example, the absence of alcohol alters the activity of brain cells, leading to unbalanced brain activity and powerful desires. In addition, adaptive changes create memories of the soothing effects of alcohol. The desire or craving can be activated by alcohol-related environmental stimuli (driving by a bar or watching TV) even after prolonged abstinence, leading to relapse. Similarly, stressful situations can trigger memories of being free from alcohol, leading to relapses.

The Mindlessness of Emotional Flooding

Detoxification is hard enough, but with initial abstinence, many issues make it challenging to focus, learn how to live a sober life, and struggle to stay clean and sober.

Before beginning treatment, many people with substance use disorders (SUDs) organize their entire daily schedule to receive, use, and recover from the effects of their addiction.

When an addict stops addictive substance or behavioral use and abuse, a gap or void exists in their daily life, and a sense of loss and grief surfaces. In grief, denial, anger, bargaining, depression, and acceptance emerge.

An emotional flood, past experiences, and trauma are associated in the early stages of grief. People in abusive or violent relationships are more likely to be emotionally flooded. Physical trauma, like the memory of injury from a car accident, can also lead to emotional flooding. A traumatic brain injury can alter moods and behaviors, leading to emotional floods.

Addicts experience confusion and disorientation from engaging in overly stimulating activities before treatment. Because their routine ends at a specialized treatment facility, early abstinence is full of anxiety, disorder, or "mindlessness." As abstinence continues, the mind clears, returning them to "mindfulness" (awareness) with the direction, support, and encouragement they need to reach treatment goals.

It is necessary to fill the gap as soon as possible to achieve a sustainable period of abstinence. All high-impact inpatient programs have a busy schedule to help build a healthy, constructive structure to replace chaotic drug-seeking activity. Order and structure help reduce the risk of relapse.

A Biblical Step 4

☑ We choose to admit to God, ourselves, and another human being the exact nature of our wrongs.

In Step Four, we must stop hiding from the truth about ourselves and our misdeeds. Only by being truthful can we experience healing (John 8:32).

The Bible Says...

"Our fathers worked with us and taught us for just a few years, to the best of their ability; but God works to heal us for eternity, that we may partake of his perfect goodness and love. No discipline or therapy is enjoyable at the time—it's painful! But if intelligently cooperated with, it results in healing of mind, development of Christlike character, and peace of heart. Therefore, stiffen your upper lip and straighten your spine, and redouble your determination to stay the healing course. 'Remove the obstacles to your recovery' so that the infection of selfishness may not permanently deform your character, but rather that you may be healed." (Hebrews 12:10-13 REM)

Phase 3: Long-term Abstinence Recovery — Sobriety is the Start of Recovery Training!

Is there a difference between sobriety and recovery? The simplest way to think of abstinence or sobriety is a sustained state of "NO" addictive substances or compulsions. Recovery is the healing and maturation of the spirit, mind, and body from enslavement. In addiction treatment, abstinence is the beginning of recovery training.

When I enlisted in the military, I learned that the foundation of basic training (boot camp) was physical and mental strength to carry out military service. Confidence and ability to make informed decisions. Advanced knowledge of survival skills such as first aid, navigation, and hand-to-hand combat. I also learned the unquestionable requirement of teamwork (Genesis 1:26-27).

Being sober is not the same as being recovered. When we think of drinking, we immediately think of abstinence from substances and compulsions. But recovery is more than behavior. It's also about mental and emotional healing.

Extended sobriety, also known as long-term abstinence, is when the addict surrenders to the admission and acceptance of a lifelong one-day-at-a-time treatment process. However, treatment and continued focus on abstinence is not enough to ensure recovery and a positive lifestyle.

The medical model calls the state of addiction a disease, and I do not dispute that. Metaphorically, think of it as a disease of selfishness that tempts us from history, from evidence and facts, and toward our insatiable inner monster, the mind & body — the flesh (Romans 8:7-8).

The flesh or addictive personality provokes strong emotions to keep the conscience from being recognized and consumed by the terrors of unremedied selfishness.

"Those who live with the selfish nature [the flesh] in charge have their minds bent on self-indulgence and selfish [flesh] pursuits; but those who live in harmony with the Spirit of truth and love have their minds focused on living in harmony with God's principles of truth, love, and liberty. The mind of the selfish [flesh] person is filled with death, but the mind governed by the principles of the Spirit of truth and love is filled with life and peace. The selfish [flesh] mind operates on the survival-of-the-fittest principle, which says, 'I love myself so much that I will kill you in order that I may live;' and such a mind is at war with the God of love, who says, 'I love you so much that I will give my life in order that you might live.' The mind of the selfish [flesh] person does not surrender to the principle of love—which requires death to self-interest—nor can it do so; those controlled by the selfish [flesh] nature cannot please God, because everything they do is opposed to all that God is." (Romans 8:5-8 REM) (emphasis mine)

In the Bible, all body parts form an entity known as "flesh," governed by sin — selfishness — where there is flesh and all forms of corruption (egoism/selfishness) where no good thing can live. Perhaps we can view the addictive personality as our inner monster, the flesh, representing our anti-God tendencies and desires in every aspect of our lives.

The disease of selfishness is the false prophet heralding the need for an authority — addiction — to believe because the leader wields a power that wows us. The combined tactics of the disease of selfishness and the God of addiction disconnect the mind from objective truth and disempower the individual from making their own informed choices, making the reason vulnerable to losing self-control and integrity. The Bible warned against this by saying:

"If a prophet, or one who foretells by dreams, appears among you and announces to you a sign or wonder, and if the sign or wonder spoken of takes place, and the prophet says, 'Let us follow other Gods" (Gods you have not known) "and let us worship them,' you must not listen to the words of that prophet or dreamer. The Lord your God is testing you to find out whether you love him with all your heart and with all your soul." (Deuteronomy 13:1–3 NIV)

In the Old Testament Book of Deuteronomy, Moses realized the pagan religions and worship of a multitude of false Gods would persist unless the people addressed the love and goodness of our creator God. Moses identifies sources leading people away from satisfaction, security, and significance. He addresses three areas:

- A false prophet leading the nation astray
- An individual leading a family astray
- Troublemakers leading a community away[114]

The false Gods are the manifestations of the disease of selfishness affecting appearance, ability, age, friends, race, gender, work, home, family, or experience.

---

[114] NIV Grace and Truth Study Bible, Deuteronomy 13:1-3, Copyright © 2021 by Zondervan. All rights reserved.

During long-term abstinence, it helps to think the disease is selfishness. The Gods can be alcoholism, substance abuse, inhalant abuse, steroid misuse, compulsive gambling, eating, video gaming, shopping, or sex.

By replacing the use or abuse of artificial highs from substances or compulsions with natural highs from activity, they may achieve sobriety but dampening recovery because they are still escaping to feel good. Remember, the four pillars of recovery are health, home, purpose, and community.

"Are you really so foolish that you think that after experiencing the healing power of the Spirit, which came by trust alone, you can now complete the healing process by your own effort—without the Spirit? Have you really gone so far in the treatment course for nothing? And it will be for nothing if you persist in trying to heal yourselves? Is it because you observe a set of rules that God enlightens your minds with his Spirit and miraculously transforms your characters, or is it because you have been won to trust by the evidence Jesus revealed?" (Galatians 3:3-5 REM)

We are people with heartaches and problems who need heart solutions. But we try to solve heart issues with intelligence, willpower, morality, and self-soothing—a pointless waste of time and energy.

Fortunately, Clinical Christian Counseling and other forms of counseling, behavioral therapies, self-help groups, and psychiatric medications tailored to specific compulsive disorders offer hope for effective treatment and recovery of any addiction.

A Biblical Step 5...

☑ We choose to accept God's grace in a relationship by being entirely ready to have God remove all these character defects.

As we confess our wickedness and experience love and acceptance from God and humans, our shame is replaced with love, which empowers us to heal. (see John 8:1-11; Jeremiah 33:8; Ezekiel 36:25-27; Hebrews 8:10)

The Bible Says...

"It is your own face that you see reflected in the water and it is your own self that you see in your heart...He [Jesus] explained further: 'What comes out of the mouth is an expression of what is in the heart — an expression of the character — and evil in the character is what makes a person impure. For evil originates from the infection of selfishness in the heart, such as evil thoughts, sexual perversity, murder, dishonesty, theft, betrayal of trust, greed, cruelty, deception, vulgarity, envy, evil-speaking, gossip, pride, and foolishness. All these destructive deviations from God's design come from inside and are what makes a person impure.'" (Proverbs 27:19 GNT; Mark 7:20-23 REM) (brackets added)

Phase 4: Continuous Recovery — *Recovery Is A New Life!*

Sobriety is an accomplishment, and recovery is a new life. The focus of recovery is not just on abstinence but on truly renewing your mind and heart to live a life of truth, love, and freedom.

Biblically speaking, restoration is an inner work that God accomplishes by the Spirit of God, convincing our hearts of truth. When we sincerely believe in His reality, the result is an effortless expression of the Fruit of His Spirit. There is no truth without evidence of the Fruit — love, joy, peace, patience, kindness, goodness, faithfulness, gentleness, and self-control (Galatians 5:22-23 NIV).

The challenge is to determine what is preventing recovery. The answer is not to try harder to believe, to control your behavior, or to do your best to live and look like Jesus. Question what you think because it dramatically impacts everything you feel and do.

If we believe a lie, it will appear valid and inevitably impede our recovery by affecting our thoughts, feelings, and behavior. However, when we know the truth about God and who we are to Him, we will be strengthened to live that truth.

When we speak of unbelief, we don't mean a person doesn't believe anything. The mind must rest on something; he clings to error when he does not grasp the truth. All people believe in some way, and their beliefs affect their hearts and character.

The fruits of the Spirit that ripen during recovery are God's Fruits, not our actions.

Performance-based recovery will never work because God didn't create the human species that way. The Fruit of the Spirit is the natural result of abiding in Christ (in the Spirit) and knowing the truth in your heart, not a list of "things to do" (Galatians 5:16-26).

The Fruit of the Spirit is God's fruit, not ours. There's a reason many people don't get the victory they hope for in recovery: doing your best wasn't the answer. "Let go, and let God!"

Until the addict understands the root cause of their addiction, they will drastically limit the benefits of learning during recovery. Sobriety stops drug use, abuse, and compulsions, and recovery matures through the lessons learned from life that lead to the Fruits of the Spirit.

"But the outgrowth of the Spirit of love is a character like God's— manifesting character traits of love, joy, peace, patience, kindness, goodness, trustworthiness, gentleness, and self-control—complete self-governance. With character like this, there is no need for a written law to diagnose defects, or quarantine, or provide external supervision, because those who have been unified with Christ Jesus have had the selfish nature with all its motives and desires eradicated from their characters. Since we are being healed by the working of the Spirit of love and truth, let us choose to cooperate with him in every way. So don't show off or try to make a name for yourself; this only tempts others to become jealous and envious, and leads their minds away from Jesus." (Galatians 5:22-26 REM)

It is impossible to fully recover if we avoid the fight by distracting ourselves from the pain. We often do this by blaming others or our circumstances for our addiction or by playing the role of victim. If we continue to avoid the truths of our lives, we lose the opportunities God has given us for our benefit and good.

There's a big difference between acting like you're getting better and "being" in recovery. Pretending is a choice to control behavior, while "being" results from the inner work of God's Spirit convincing us of the truth in our hearts.

Suppressing what we think or feel in an attempt to "obey" God can bring temporary relief, but such controlled behavior is neither spiritual nor authentic to recovery. Also, coping with pain based on lies is neither spiritual nor indicates whether a person is recovering well (James 4:7-10).

"Surrender yourselves to God and his treatment. Tell the devil No, and you will escape him. Move close to God, and God will come close to you. You selfish people! Stop choosing to indulge your desires. Stop going back and forth between love and selfishness, and purify your hearts with love. Stop playing around and get real! Let your hearts break: Cry over your terminal condition, admit that you are sick, and stop pretending that all is well. Then go humbly to the Lord, and he will heal and restore you." (James 4:7-10 REM)

Recovery is the process of growing in our heart's beliefs about how we live that are larger than what we intellectually hold to be true. Intellectual ideas help us navigate our day-to-day affairs. Still, our heartfelt beliefs determine how we perceive ourselves (self-identity) and our current situation, which expresses our view of God's participation in our life (state of being).

"Intellectual belief helps us know what to do, but heart belief produces the motivating forces behind what I do (whether good or not). In those times in which our heart-belief is contrary to the truth that we know intellectually, the heart will always win out (even when I believe the truth intellectually). However, if we are "renewed in the spirit of your mind" (Ephesians 4:23) —the renewal of our Heart Belief— genuine change will be made manifest by the effortless transformation expressed by the natural outflow and bearing of the Spirit's fruit (Romans 12:2)." (Smith, E., 2019)[115]

Biblical perfection is not about behavior. But the biblical ideal is about the maturation of the heart attitude, where we come to love God and other's more than we love ourselves.

Continued participation in counseling, group, family, and 12-step programs is crucial in maintaining long-term abstinence and

[115] Smith, E. (2019) Retrieved from https://www.transformationprayer.org/wp-content/uploads/2019/12/Process-of-TPM-Dec-2019.pdf. —15

recovery. Accepting that addiction is chronic, progressive, incurable, and potentially fatal helps obstruct the possibility of relapse.

Dr. Darryl Inaba (1997) tells us that addiction is incurable. He states, "Can we cure addiction? Not! Addiction causes unrecoverable changes, alterations, and death of brain cells. Brain cells are not readily regenerated like other cells, so the change is caused by drug abuse or permanent. What we can do is arrest the illness, teach new living techniques, rewire the brain to bypass those addicted cells, and help an addict in recovery live a worthwhile life. Although addiction cannot be cured, it can be effectively prevented and treated."[116]

Substance use disorders can have severe consequences for the functioning of the entire nervous system, especially the brain. These effects include changes in emotions and personality and impairments in cognition, learning, and memory.[117]

SPECT brain scans vividly illustrate the harmful effects of toxic exposure to drugs and alcohol. These addictive substances detrimentally affect critical regions of the brain, which are essential for optimizing your overall well-being and quality of life. To see the effects of drugs and alcohol on the brain, see the brain scans for yourself at https://www.amenclinics.com/ blog/10-ways-brain-scanscan-help-with-addictions/.

Direct self-control practice (i.e., small acts of impulse control, such as avoiding candy, practiced for two weeks before quitting) significantly improved abstinence rates in cigarette smokers; 27% of participants assigned to self-management training, compared to 12% of participants in the control group, were still abstaining one month after quitting.[118]

Successful training to control cognitive cravings through Cognitive Behavioral Therapy reflects on the long-term effects of drug-related visual cues. The movement has also demonstrated increased prefrontal cortex activity and down-regulate corpus striatum activity in the brain.[119]

Research indicates that successful abstinence is greatly enhanced

---

[116] Ibid. Inaba (1997)
[117] https://www.ncbi.nlm.nih.gov/pmc/articles/PMC6826797/
[118] https://www.ncbi.nlm.nih.gov/pmc/articles/PMC3706547/
[119] Ibid. Inaba.

by retraining the mind and body—spirit, soul, and body. To a Christian Counselor, Cognitive Behavioral Therapy (CBT) is a secularized Biblical Counseling model that emphasizes right over wrong thinking.

Throughout His ministry, Jesus consistently emphasized to the disciples that it was their responsibility to work alongside Him to free the world from sin's bondage. He demonstrated this by sending out the Twelve and later the Seventy to proclaim the gospel of the kingdom of God, instructing them to share what He had taught them with others.

Jesus' ministry served as a training ground for the disciples to learn how to work independently and to gradually expand their efforts to reach all corners of the earth. His final message to His followers was that they held a crucial role in spreading the message of salvation to the rest of the world. Disseminating the good news was their duty and responsibility.

A Biblical Step 7

☑ Made a list of all persons we had harmed and became willing to make amends to them all.

The seventh step involves recognizing our inability to alter our personalities or inherent qualities and seeking God's transformative power through daily communication with Him.

The Bible Says...

"So if you are presenting your offering at the altar, and while there you remember that your brother has something [such as a grievance or legitimate complaint] against you, leave your offering there at the altar and go. First make peace with your brother, and then come and present your offering." (Matthew 5:23-24 AMP)

CHAPTER 13

UNMASKING RELAPSE PREVENTION

RELAPSE PREVENTION — *Not Letting The Past Steal Your Present!*

It is essential to focus on the present and not allow past failures to hinder progress toward recovery. Experts in addictions acknowledge that people often seek treatment to prevent relapse due to their prior unsuccessful efforts to overcome their addictive behaviors or substance abuse.

Relapse is an essential aspect of addiction and presents itself in two ways. Firstly, there are addictive behaviors and chemical dependence signs that manifest during periods of active use. Secondly, symptoms occur during abstinence, which creates a tendency toward relapse and becomes an integral part of the illness.

Relapse entails a regression towards non-functional states due to sobriety-based symptoms that can lead to renewed addictive behavior, drug or alcohol consumption, emotional or physical collapse, or even suicide. Identifying warning signs that appear well before relapse helps predict the process.

Recovery is a progression of personal development with specific milestones. Each step of recovery carries its risks of relapse.

Most of the time, relapse occurs gradually, allowing you to break it down into distinct phases. Treatment for relapse prevention aims to aid individuals in identifying the initial stages of deterioration when the probability of success is higher.

To develop effective coping mechanisms, the critical tools for relapse prevention include cognitive therapy that involves recognizing and replacing negative thought patterns, gaining spiritual knowledge, and using mind-body relaxation techniques.

Counselors help individuals who are struggling with relapse by teaching them to recognize and manage these signs and to interrupt the process early, thereby facilitating a return to positive progress in recovery.

To possess courage does not necessarily mean having the physical or emotional power to persist; courage carries on even when you feel depleted of any strength.

Five Primary Goals of Relapse Prevention

Prevention is a thorough approach to stop clients who suffer from behavioral or chemical dependence from relapsing into addictive behavior.[120]

1. Assess the global lifestyle patterns contributing to relapse by completing a comprehensive self-assessment of life, addiction, and history.

2. Construct a personalized list of warning signs that lead the relapse from stable recovery to chemical use.

3. Develop warning sign management strategies for the critical warning signs.

4. Develop a structured recovery program that will allow clients to identify and manage the critical warning signs as they occur.

5. Develop a relapse early intervention plan to provide the client and significant others with step-by-step instructions to interrupt alcohol and other drug use should it recur.

---

[120] Gorski, T.T., and Miller, M. (1986) *Staying Sober: A Guide for Relapse Prevention.* Independence, MO: Herald House/Independence Press.

Six Stages of Recovery

The recovery, or as some have called it, healing, involves six stages in which individuals gradually develop healthy habits. The first stage, known as *Transition*, requires the recognition of addiction and the desire to achieve abstinence. The second stage, *Stabilization*, involves stabilizing one's psychosocial life crisis and recovering from acute and post-acute withdrawal from drugs or alcohol. *Early recovery*, the third stage, entails identifying and replacing addictive thoughts, feelings, and behaviors with those prioritizing sobriety. The fourth stage, *Middle Recovery*, involves repairing lifestyle damage caused by addiction and establishing a balanced, healthy lifestyle. *Late Recovery*, the fifth stage, deals with resolving family-of-origin issues that can lead to relapse. Finally, in the *Maintenance* stage, clients continue to grow and maintain an active recovery program to avoid slipping back into old habits.[121]

In relapse prevention, to achieve a healthy and balanced state of recovery, the processes involve addressing the biological, psychological, and social aspects of the individual experiencing addiction — biopsychosocial (BPS). These elements consider three primary psychological domains (Thinking, Feeling, and Acting) and three primary social domains (Work, Acquaintances, and Close Personal Relationships).

In this model, each domain is equally important. The aim is to enable clients to attain competent functioning in these domains. In most cases, clients prefer one psychological and one social part, which can lead to an overdeveloped state in these areas while others remain underdeveloped.

The goal is to reinforce skills in the overdeveloped domains while building up skills in the underdeveloped ones, thus achieving a more balanced and healthy functioning.

A Healthy Brain Strengthens Relapse Prevention

The BPS model acknowledges that both addictive behaviors and chemical addiction can lead to changes in brain function. Behaviors

---

[121] Ibid. Gorski

that are addictive stimulate reward systems in a way similar to the stimulation caused by drug abuse — anticipation completion. These behaviors also produce some behavioral symptoms identical to those observed in people suffering from substance use disorders.

It also recognizes addiction as a primary illness that results in abusing addictive behaviors or mood-altering substances. Prolonged use of these behaviors or substances can cause brain dysfunction, resulting in a disorganized personality and difficulties in social and occupational settings.

Complete recovery requires eliminating addictive behaviors or substance use and significantly changing one's personality and way of living.

Individuals who grow up in troubled families may develop self-sabotaging behavior patterns (as early as 2 to 4), referred to as character defects by AA, that hinder their ability to overcome addiction. Because addiction is a chronic illness, relapse is a common occurrence.

Relapse can lead to dysfunction during recovery, culminating in physical or emotional breakdowns, self-medication with substances, or suicide. Recovery addresses issues related to brain dysfunction, personality fragmentation, social dysfunction, and familial conflict, all of which contribute to relapse and recovery challenges.

The relapse syndrome is a fundamental aspect of the addictive disease process, consisting of obsessive desires or drug-related symptoms during abstinence. These sobriety-based symptoms contribute to a bias towards relapse inherent in the disease.

Relapse occurs when individuals become impaired in their sobriety due to these symptoms, resulting in renewed substance use, physical or emotional deterioration, or even suicide.

Recognizable warning signs precede the relapse process, providing opportunities for individuals to interrupt the progression and return to a path of positive progress in recovery. Recovery counseling educates clients on identifying and managing these warning signs effectively.

Brain dysfunction can occur in several stages of addiction, including periods of intoxication short-term and long-term withdrawal. Individuals with a genetic predisposition to addiction seem more vulnerable to this brain dysfunction. As the addiction progresses, the symptoms of this brain dysfunction can affect cognitive ability, emotional management, memory, sleep, stress management, and coordination.

The symptoms can be most severe during the first 6 to 18 months of sobriety, and their recurrence may occur during physical or psychosocial stress, even in the long run.

The disruption of normal cognitive, emotional, and behavioral processes in the brain leads to personality disorganization. While some instances are temporary and can resolve as the brain heals, others may become entrenched due to prolonged addiction and require professional intervention. Social issues such as family, employment, legal matters, and finances may arise due to this brain dysfunction and subsequent personality disorganization.

The development of addiction is not the direct cause of self-defeating personality traits. The developing years within a dysfunctional family influence negative character development. We are birthed with a combination of dominant Temperament and Personality, starting in DNA, developing through childhood interactions, and continuing unconsciously into adulthood (Psalm 139).

Our Temperament and Personality become a habitual way of thinking, feeling, acting, and relating to others, nurtured by genetics and interactions with family and environment.

However, self-defeating personality traits and disorders can exacerbate the progression, identification, and treatment of addiction and increase the risk of relapse. It is essential, therefore, to address family-of-origin issues appropriately in addiction treatment.

"You created every part of me; you put me together in my mother's womb. I praise you because you are to be feared; all you do is strange and wonderful. I know it with all my heart. When my bones were being formed, carefully put together in my mother's womb, when I was growing there in secret, you knew that I was there—you saw me before I was born. The days allotted to me had all been recorded in your book, before any of them ever began." (Psalms 139:13-16 GNT)

Clients recovering from addiction and learning to avoid relapse can find comfort in knowing God has been committed to them even before birth. God watched over them while they were in their mother's womb, fortifying and guiding them until they were born. We are all uniquely crafted, and the word "fearfully" in this context means admiring our bodies' complexity. This information can be helpful for those going through recovery and relapse prevention.

God created our physical bodies and lives, including every day ordained for us. Therefore, nothing can take HIM by surprise. The psalmist's apprehension of God's infinite knowledge changes into wonder at God's concern for him.

We also can feel secure knowing that God loves us more than our parents. Describing God's thoughts is impractical, as it is comparable to counting each grain of sand: *"How precious to me are your thoughts, O God! How vast is the sum of them!"* (Psalms 139:17 GNT) — Thoughts of me and you.

A Biblical Step 8 & 9

☑ We continued to take personal inventory and, when we were
   wrong, promptly admitted it.

To put it differently, in steps eight and nine, we implement fresh approaches, values, and intentions in our lives by regularly examining ourselves and admitting our mistakes. This entails prioritizing the well-being and health of others over our interests, allowing us to progress toward God's healing and liberation.[122]

The Bible Says...

So be sure to admit to one another where you have deviated from God's design, and request God's intervention and treatment plan for each other, so that you may be healed. The request of a person who lives in unity with God is powerful and effective.
(James 5:16 REM)

---

[122] Jennings, T., (2009) "Biblical Approach To Addictions," https://comeandreason.com/biblical-approach-to-addictions3/

CHAPTER 14

EMPOWERING TOGETHER —
UNVEILING THE COLLECTIVE PATH TO
ADDICTION RECOVERY SUCCESS!

Let's explore ways to stay connected to your addiction support network during these unprecedented times. Relapse rates for addictive behaviors and substance use disorders are high, but it is possible to prevent them from happening.

Addictive behaviors and Substance use disorders can be challenging to overcome, but they are not impossible. Seeking and completing treatment is an essential step in recovery, but it is not the end. One of the main concerns for anyone in recovery is relapse.

Among the treatment goals are to help individuals recognize the early warning signs of relapse and develop coping skills to prevent relapse early when the chances of success are most significant.

Relapse rates for addictive behaviors and substance use disorders are high, but it is possible to prevent it from happening. The following are some tips for avoiding substance use disorder relapse.

Staying Connected to Your Addiction Support Network

Recovery is not a solo journey. It is essential to build a support network that is available when you need it. Stay connected with your sponsor, counselor, and sober friends. They can offer support, motivation, and accountability during your recovery journey.

Addiction can be a tough challenge to overcome. It is essential to have a robust support system in place to help stay on track towards recovery. We've learned from the alleged COVID-19 pandemic staying connected to your addiction support network has become more challenging than ever.

Let's explore ways to stay connected to your addiction support network during these unprecedented times.

1. Virtual support groups: Many addiction support groups have shifted to virtual meetings using video conferencing tools like Zoom and Skype. These digital platforms offer a way to connect without leaving your home. Contact your support group to determine if they have moved to virtual meetings and how to join their online sessions.

2. Tele-counseling: With the increased attention on social distancing, some addiction treatment centers have started offering tele-counseling services. These services allow individuals to talk to addiction professionals from the comfort of their own homes. Ask your treatment center if they provide tele-counseling services and how to get started.

3. Conference calls: With the rise of digital tools, conference calls can be a valuable way to connect with your support network. Set up a conference call with your family, friends, or support group. This will allow you to check in with each other and offer support without physically being present, as well as "Group Me" texting.

4. Online forums: Many online forums are dedicated to addiction recovery. These forums offer a chance to share experiences and offer support to others. Joining an online forum can be a great way to connect with others who understand your struggles.

   Online forums are virtual gathering places on the Internet, enabling individuals to engage in meaningful dialogues. Unlike chat rooms, which feature rapid message exchanges, these forums facilitate gradual conversations. Furthermore, they differ from social media platforms, often centering around specific topics, brands, or fan communities.

An example of an Online Forum for Addictions is https://www.reddit.com/r/addictions/.

5. Self-care: Self-care is essential to addiction recovery. Make sure to take care of your physical and mental health. This includes eating healthy foods, regular exercise, and getting enough sleep.

The current era tends to overlook a significant problem in addiction recovery: loneliness. It is considered a severe epidemic that affects people across the globe, and the United States is no exception. As per a recent survey, approximately 75% of Americans experience loneliness, while reports from Forbes reveal that the number of people encountering isolation has risen three times over the past 40 years. This issue is undoubtedly concerning, and as followers of the Christian faith, we should do our part in showing compassion toward those who feel lonely.[123] [124]

The alleged COVID-19 pandemic has brought new challenges to addiction recovery. However, it is essential to remember that there are ways to stay connected to your addiction support network; be prepared for the next time. Whether through virtual support groups, tele-counseling services, conference calls, or online forums, you can stay connected and get the help and support you need.

A Biblical Step 10

☑ Through prayer and meditation, we sought to improve our conscious contact with God as we understood Him, praying only for knowledge of His Will for us and the power to carry that out.

---

[123] Retrieved from https://www.prnewswire.com/news-releases/survey-finds-nearly-three-quarters-72-of-americans-feel-lonely-300342742.html

[124] Retrieved from https://www.forbes.com/sites/carolinebeaton/2017/02/09/why-millennials-are-lonely/?sh=29aa7e057c35

A Scriptural Step 10 safeguards against the formation of new errors, ensuring they do not evolve into entrenched habits.

The Bible Says...

"Therefore arm your minds with God's full set of armor so that when Satan's grand deception comes and it seems the heavens are about to fall, you are able to stand; and when you have done everything to present the truth and expose Satan's lies [addiction's lies]–don't falter; stand! Stand firm, with the truth of God wrapped around you like a belt; with a righteous, Christlike character developed within–like a breastplate; and the peace that comes from accepting the good news about God–like track shoes providing good traction and a solid foundation. Also, hold fast the shield of trust, which extinguishes all the burning fear and insecurity brought by the devil's [addiction's] temptations. Take with you the helmet of a healed mind–a mind protected from the assaults of Satan; and attack the lies about God with the sword of the Spirit, which is the word of God–the truth. And talk with God with an enlightened mind, intelligently, on all occasions, about all of your concerns, requests, plans, and issues. With all of this in mind, be alert and always keep praying for God's people."(Ephesians 6:13-18 REM)

CHAPTER 15

UNDERSTANDING ADDICTION RELAPSE TRIGGERS

Individuals can enhance their chances of maintaining long-term recovery by identifying and addressing relapse triggers of high-risk situations, emotional triggers, social pressure, overconfidence and complacency, negative or distorted thinking patterns, celebratory or triggering events, and physical discomfort or pain.

Addiction is a disease that affects millions of individuals every year, and unfortunately, there is no cure for it. However, the treatment available can help individuals manage their addiction and achieve long-term recovery. Even with successful treatment and recovery, relapse is always a possibility.

Understanding addiction relapse triggers is indeed crucial in preventing relapse from occurring. Relapse or regression refers to a return to substance abuse or addictive behaviors after abstinence or recovery. It can be a challenging and disheartening experience for individuals seeking to overcome addiction.

Here are some common catalysts that frequently result in a recurrence of addiction:

High-Risk Situations:

High-risk situations for addiction are circumstances or conditions that may trigger a craving or relapse in someone trying to overcome or manage substance use or behavioral addiction. The cues of certain people, places, or things associated with past substance use or addictive behavior can trigger cravings. These situations are typically associated with the specific addiction the person is dealing with and can vary significantly from person to person.

Certain high-risk situations can increase the chances of a relapse in your journey towards recovery. It's essential to be aware of these situations and take precautions to avoid them. Some of these high-risk situations include being in the presence of substances, being around people who use drugs or engage in addictive behaviors, or visiting places associated with past substance abuse. Avoiding such environments and seeking support from your loved ones and professional counselors is crucial.

Emotional triggers:

As individuals, we may experience a variety of emotional states, such as stress, anxiety, depression, anger, loneliness, or boredom, which can excite the urge to turn to substance abuse as a way of coping. These emotional triggers may exert significant influence, so developing more beneficial coping strategies to overcome them is essential.

In moments of transition or change, emotional triggers can frequently arise. Significant life events, like relocation, embarking on a new career, or terminating a relationship, can generate stress and uncertainty. Consequently, individuals may attempt to cope with these emotions through substance consumption or addictive actions. Additionally, facing interpersonal conflicts can be emotionally arduous, causing some people to turn to substances or addictive behaviors to seek relief or diversion.

Social pressure:

Social pressure is the influence that peers, acquaintances, or family members who continue to engage in addictive behavior can have and represent a significant trigger for a relapse. Attending events where substances are freely available or the addictive behavior is normalized can be high-risk. Creating a robust and supportive group of individuals wholeheartedly dedicated to recovery is crucial. Parents may have to help their teenagers develop new social groups.

Overconfidence and complacency:

Experiencing an exaggerated confidence or contentment regarding one's recovery can decrease attentiveness. Overconfident or complacent persons will test willpower or personal control, placing them in high-risk situations where they previously used a substance or engaged in addictive behavior.

A mindset like this could cause individuals to believe they can engage in behaviors or substance abuse without facing the consequences, ultimately returning to previous negative states. Remaining alert to vulnerabilities demonstrates the importance of staying watchful and grounded to prevent the dangers of excessive confidence.

Negative or distorted thinking patterns:

Unproductive thoughts, lack of self-confidence, impractical convictions, or distorted thought processes can impede rehabilitation endeavors. Typical illustrations comprise "I have already ruined everything, therefore, might as well continue utilizing" or "I can handle my addiction this moment."

Celebratory or triggering events:

Regarding substance abuse, certain events such as special occasions, celebrations, holidays, or significant life moments can potentially trigger a relapse. Just as negative emotions can trigger substance use, so can positive ones. Festivals, parties, or other joyful events can lead to substance use or a return to addictive behaviors.

These events frequently include social gatherings where substances may be easily accessible, and the urge to celebrate or deal with emotions can pose a relapse hazard. It's essential to be mindful of these risks and take necessary precautions to maintain sobriety during such occasions.

Physical discomfort or pain:

Feelings of physical unease or agony: Undergoing chronic pain, physical discomfort, or sickness can trigger a relapse. One may feel compelled to use substances to alleviate discomfort or avoid suffering.

Recognizing circumstances with a heightened potential for relapse is essential to overcoming addiction and steering clear of setbacks. Professionals such as therapists and counselors consistently collaborate with individuals to assist them in pinpointing their unique high-risk situations. Together, they devise effective strategies to manage and navigate these situations while fostering personal strength and resilience to minimize their influence. Doing so will empower individuals to withstand the temptations and triggers that may hinder their recovery journey and can lead them astray.

Your Cliff Notes to Addiction Recovery and Relapse Prevention

To prevent relapse, it's crucial to develop effective relapse-prevention strategies, such as:

- Building a solid support system: Surround yourself with supportive and understanding individuals committed to your recovery. A robust support system can significantly improve your mental health, resilience, and overall quality of life. Whether it's family, friends, coworkers, mentors, or professional therapists and counselors, the people in your support system can provide emotional assistance, guidance, and different perspectives. It's okay to lean on your support system. It's what they're there for. Asking for help is not a sign of weakness but a sign of strength, as it shows you understand your own needs and limits.

- Developing healthy coping mechanisms: It is imperative to cultivate constructive strategies for dealing with cravings and stress, conquering obstacles, and successfully navigating the rollercoaster of life. This crucial aspect of personal development enables individuals to manage their emotions effectively and achieve overall well-being. Much like the wisdom found in the Bible, developing resilient coping mechanisms provides valuable insights and motivation, encouraging individuals to rise above adversity and find inspiration amidst life's uncertainties. Thus, by embracing healthy strategies for managing stress, one can attain clarity of mind and successfully navigate life's ups and downs.

- Identifying and avoiding triggers: Triggers encompass various stimuli that can evoke intense emotions, typically of a negative nature, in individuals. These stimuli can be associated with many issues, such as traumatic experiences, mental health disorders, addictions, etc. Recognizing that triggers are subjective and can differ significantly from one person to another is crucial. In the realm of human emotions, it is entirely natural and beneficial to experience various emotional reactions. There is no shame in feeling upset or stressed from time to time. However, the ultimate objective in identifying and evading triggers is not to evade all negative emotions altogether. Instead, it enhances our ability to regulate and comprehend our emotional responses, preventing them from overpowering or dictating our lives. This approach, grounded in professionalism and biblical principles, aims to provide wisdom, motivation, and clarity, serving as an inspiration to lead a well-managed, fulfilling existence.

- Seeking professional help: Engage in ongoing therapy, counseling, or support groups to address underlying issues, develop relapse prevention skills, and gain additional support. They seek the assistance of experts in a specific field who express a tone of professionalism with a biblical and Christian perspective to provide insightful and motivating guidance. Good leaders, therapists, counselors, and coaches will utilize persuasive techniques through references, inspiration, and clarity.

- Taking care of your physical and mental health: In today's fast-paced world, it is crucial to prioritize the respect of both our physical and mental health. As followers of Christ, one call is to steward our bodies as temples of the Holy Spirit (1 Corinthians 6:19). By nurturing our physical and mental well-being, we better equip ourselves to fulfill God's purpose. Caring for our physical health goes beyond simply exercising and eating well. It involves recognizing that our bodies are a precious gift from God and treating them with the respect and honor they deserve. Regular exercise, balanced nutrition, and sufficient rest are essential to maintain physical strength and vitality.

- Similarly, tending to our mental health is vital for our overall well-being. There is an intricate connection between our spiritual and emotional health. The Bible encourages us to guard our minds and fill them with thoughts that are proper, honorable, just, pure, lovely, commendable, and praiseworthy (Philippians 4:8). Practice self-care by prioritizing sleep, maintaining a healthy diet, exercising regularly, and seeking treatment for any co-occurring mental health conditions.

- Developing a relapse prevention plan: Work with professionals to create a personalized relapse prevention plan that outlines strategies, coping mechanisms, and steps to take in case of a relapse—developing a strategy to avoid deterioration in one's life journey. This plan incorporates a professional and inspiring tone, drawing wisdom from the Bible and Christian teachings. It aims to provide insightful and motivating references while ensuring clarity and a persuasive approach.

Do not view relapse as a failure in the journey toward recovery. Instead, see it as an integral part of the process. With the appropriate support and strategies, individuals can gain valuable insights from their relapse and use them to further their pursuit of long-term sobriety and well-being. By staying motivated, seeking guidance from trusted sources, and applying the lessons learned, one can continue on a path of healing and transformation. Through this lens, you are transforming relapse into a stepping stone toward personal growth and a testament to the resilience of the human spirit.

It's crucial to maintain awareness that there are healthier coping mechanisms that can help you manage these emotions. As a Christian Counselor, I believe that turning to God and HIS Word can be a powerful tool for managing emotional triggers. Reading the Bible, praying, and seeking guidance from Christian Counselors and leaders can provide comfort and support during difficult times.

How To Feel Better In Less Than Twelve Minutes

In addition to spiritual support, you can also take practical steps to develop healthier coping mechanisms. These may include exercise, meditation, mindfulness practices, or seeking professional help such as counseling or therapy.

Take Deep Breaths (2 minutes): Start by doing deep breathing for 2 minutes. Deep breaths can help you calm your nervous system and ease stress.

Hydrate (1 minute): Drink a glass of water. Dehydration can cause feelings of anxiety and make you feel low.

Move Your Body (3 minutes): Do a mini workout, stretch, or go for a short walk. This can release endorphins, which are natural mood lifters.

Gratitude (2 minutes): Write three things you're grateful for. Research has shown that practicing gratitude can significantly improve your mood and happiness.

Mindful Biblical Meditation (2 minutes): Take the time to reflect on a specific Bible verse, centering your attention on your breath and releasing any extraneous thoughts. Direct your focus solely on the message God intends for you to derive from the verse while remaining fully present in the current moment. Embrace the relevance of the scripture in your present circumstances, allowing it to inspire and motivate you on your Christian journey.

Positive Affirmations (1 minute): Look in the mirror and tell yourself some positive affirmations. It might feel silly, but it can powerfully impact your mood and self-esteem.

Laugh (1 minute): Watch a funny video or think about a funny moment from your past. Laughter can be a great stress reliever.

This daily practice may not offer lasting solutions to enduring challenges or deeply rooted emotional issues. Yet, it can provide immediate comfort during moments of distress or anxiety. It is important to remember that seeking professional assistance is acceptable if you consistently experience sadness or if your emotional state interferes with your daily activities. As Christians, we can find inspiration and motivation in biblical references that guide us toward seeking help and finding solace in challenging times.

Remembering that you are not alone in your struggle with addiction relapse triggers is essential. You can overcome these challenges and lead a healthy, fulfilling life with the proper support and tools.

A Biblical Step 11

☑ Having had a spiritual awakening due to these steps, we tried to carry this message to alcoholics and to practice these principles in all our affairs.

The eleventh step entails enhancing our communion with God, promoting the development of new, health-giving neural pathways that eventually rewire our neurological framework over a prolonged period.[125]

The Bible Says...

Those who live with the selfish nature in charge have their minds bent on self-indulgence and selfish pursuits; but those who live in harmony with the Spirit of truth and love have their minds focused on living in harmony with God's principles of truth, love, and liberty. The mind of the selfish person is filled with death, but the mind governed by the principles of the Spirit of truth and love is filled with life and peace. (Romans 8:5-6 REM)

---

[125] *file:///Usrs/pierresamaan/Documents/My Files/SubstDis/JENNINGS/Biblical Approach to Addictions.html

CHAPTER 16

INTERNAL WARNING
SIGNS OF ADDICTION

In seeking addiction recovery, being vigilant and aware of the warning signs that could hinder your progress is crucial. Maintain your course by recognizing the subsequent indications that may undermine your efforts to avoid relapse: *internal warning signs, avoidance & defensive behavior, crisis building, immobilization, confusion & overreaction, depression, behavioral loss of control, recognition of loss of control, option reduction, and return to use — physical/emotional collapse.*

This guidance aims to shed light on these indicators, drawing inspiration from biblical and Christian principles while motivating and persuading you to stay on the path of recovery. By referencing relevant sources, we provide valuable insights and guidance to keep you inspired and determined to overcome addiction.

Internal Warning Signs of Addiction Relapse

Clouded Thinking

Clouded thinking or cognitive haze is an internal indicator of a potential return to addictive behaviors. Mental haze, also known as brain fog, is not a medical condition per se but a symptom of other possible conditions. It's a feeling of being somewhat detached or disconnected from reality, as if you're in a constant state of fuzziness or haze. Clouded thinking may lead to issues with memory, concentration, focus, and the ability to perform tasks.

Regard this phenomenon as an exemplary signal in the journey of addiction recovery. A clear mind is essential, emphasizing the need for mental clarity and rational decision-making. Acknowledging this vital discernment encourages individuals to remain steadfast in overcoming addiction.

In 1 Peter 1:13 (REM), we read, *"Therefore, prepare your minds to think, to reason, to weigh out the issues, and actively apply the truth to your lives, attaining self-governance–control over your own selves. Keep your vision, goals, and hopes fixed on the full healing and restoration that will occur when Jesus Christ comes again."* Drawing wisdom from biblical teachings and relying on Christian principles, let us find inspiration to persevere and empower ourselves toward a life free from the chains of addiction.

Emotional Dysregulation

Emotional dysregulation or struggling to regulate emotions and manage feelings can be a significant clue, suggesting a possible relapse into addictive behaviors. Emotional dysregulation is a term used in the mental health community to refer to an emotional response that is poorly modulated and does not fall within the conventionally accepted range of emotive responses. It is often associated with an experience of emotional responses that are excessively intense relative to the situation at hand.

Controlling our emotions and managing our feelings can often be challenging, especially for those on the path to recovery from addiction. The healing process and moving forward is not always smooth, and relapses can indicate unresolved emotional turmoil. One of the key aspects of prevention lies in understanding our mood swings and recognizing their triggers. By delving deep into the roots of our emotions, we can unveil the underlying pain and past traumas that fuel our addiction.

Drawing inspiration from the wisdom found in the Bible, we can find solace in knowing that we are not alone in our struggles. The scripture reminds us that we can find the power to overcome our most significant challenges through God's strength. We can develop healthier coping mechanisms and build resilience by seeking guidance and relying on a solid support system. Your recovery is not defined by setbacks but rather by the courage and determination you display in the face of them. Stay committed, stay hopeful, and trust in the path that leads you to a life of emotional healing and true freedom.

Memory Troubles

Memory troubles or forgetfulness can serve as a crucial indicator of the potential of returning to addictions. As individuals embark on the recovery journey, they must be vigilant and proactive in preventing relapses. The link between memory and addiction has been well-documented in various studies, emphasizing the significant impact that memory deficits can have on one's recovery process.

Excessive use of alcohol and drugs can damage the brain and lead to memory loss, which can become a relapse agent during recovery. Some contributing factors to memory impairment are age, stress, health conditions, substance history, lack of sleep, and lack of routine. By understanding this connection, individuals can implement effective strategies to safeguard against relapse and ensure long-term sobriety.

As the Bible reminds us, *"No matter how often honest people fall, they always get up again; but disaster destroys the wicked."* (Proverbs 24:16 GNT) Let this be our inspiration to persevere through the challenges, find solace in our faith, and tap into the collective wisdom of our Christian community. Together, we can overcome the shackles of addiction and reclaim the vibrant lives God has intended for us. Let us embrace this opportunity for growth, drawing strength from our shared experiences and empowering each other along this transformative recovery journey.

Poor Stress Management

Poor stress management can serve as a potential indicator of returning to addictions. In the recovery journey, individuals battling addiction must remain vigilant in preventing relapse. Often regarded as a triggering factor, stress can exacerbate the desire to revert to old habits. Thus, it becomes imperative to cultivate effective stress management techniques.

As a Christian, one can draw inspiration from the Bible, which offers insightful teachings on managing stress. Philippians 4:6-7 (REM) states, *"You don't need to worry or fret about anything: with a thankful heart, just talk to God about all your concerns, troubles and stresses, and God's peace — that is beyond words and human explanation — will fill your minds and strengthen your hearts as you trust totally in Christ Jesus."* This scripture encourages individuals to turn to God in times of stress, finding solace in prayer and gratitude.

Additionally, seeking support from various resources such as counseling, Biblical meditation, and exercise can significantly aid in managing stress and maintaining a solid recovery. By taking proactive steps to manage stress, one can break free from the grasp of addiction and embrace a fulfilling, sober life.

Sleep Disturbances

Insomnia, or sleep disturbances, is a crucial indicator that one may be on the verge of relapsing in their battle against addiction. Understanding the interconnectedness between sleep and recovery is vital in prevention and long-term sobriety. Insomnia is a common sleep disorder characterized by difficulties falling asleep, staying asleep, waking up too early, or experiencing non-restorative sleep for at least three nights a week for a month or more, leading to daytime impairments or distress.

Studies have shown that a lack of quality sleep can lead to heightened cravings and a weakened ability to resist temptations, making it more challenging to maintain the path of recovery. Therefore, addressing and managing sleep disturbances becomes paramount in the journey towards a healthier, addiction-free life. By improving sleep hygiene, incorporating relaxation techniques, and seeking professional help, individuals can overcome insomnia and take significant strides toward sustained recovery.

Proverbs 3:24 (NIV) states, *"When you lie down, you will not be afraid; when you lie down, your sleep will be sweet."* This scripture reminds us of the divine promise of peaceful rest, reinforcing the importance of prioritizing healthy sleep patterns to overcome addiction.

Clumsiness & Disorientation

Clumsiness or being careless in physical movements can serve as a potential indicator of relapse in addiction recovery. While it may seem trivial, this lack of coordination can point to a deeper issue. Lack of coordination can be caused by neurological conditions, physical conditions, developmental delays, or brain chemistry dysregulation due to cravings. Alcohol, recreational drugs, or certain medications can impact coordination, leading to clumsiness. Impaired coordination can become a connecting agent of withdrawals or cravings during recovery.

Just as the Bible calls us to be vigilant and disciplined in all areas of our lives, it is crucial to maintain a heightened level of self-awareness and mindfulness during the recovery journey. Disorientation and clumsiness can signal a drift away from the path of long-term sobriety, reminding us that prevention is critical. By recognizing the significance of these physical manifestations, individuals can take proactive steps to address the underlying emotional, mental, or spiritual challenges they might be facing.

Let us draw inspiration from the profound transformation experienced by those who have fought addiction, using their stories as references to stay motivated and committed to our recovery. May we be encouraged to cultivate disciplined habits, engage in self-reflection, seek support from a strong community, and pursue a deeper connection with a higher power?

Intense Negative Emotions

Intense negative emotions can serve as a potential indicator of an impending relapse into addiction. Intense negative emotions are powerful feelings that can evoke considerable distress. Such emotions include fear, sadness, anger, guilt, disgust, shame, etc. While it's normal to experience a range of negative emotions in response to different life events, persistent or excessively intense negative emotions can interfere with the daily functioning of recovery and well-being.

Like all emotions, negative ones serve a purpose by signaling that something isn't right and needs our attention. However, when these emotions are intense and sustained, they can lead to significant distress and impairment, potentially resulting in conditions like anxiety disorders, depression, post-traumatic stress disorder (PTSD), and other mental health conditions.

In the recovery journey, it is essential to recognize and address these emotions with utmost diligence and care. When individuals experience intense emotions like hysteria, agitations, or rage, it is crucial to understand that these feelings often emerge due to unresolved internal conflicts or external stressors — look for reminders of past negative strongholds/traumas (a function of Complex PTSD). By acknowledging and identifying these emotions, individuals can gain valuable insights into their triggers and work towards developing healthier coping mechanisms.

Let go and let God! Drawing inspiration from biblical teachings reminds us of the importance of seeking support from a higher power and relying on a solid support network. We read in 2 Timothy 1:7 (AMP), *"For God did not give us a spirit of timidity or cowardice or fear, but [He has given us a spirit] of power and of love and of sound judgment and personal discipline [abilities that result in a calm, well-balanced mind and self-control]."* Utilizing these resources, individuals can effectively navigate the tumultuous waves of intense emotions and prevent the temptation of returning to the chains of addiction. Remember, true strength lies in confronting these emotions and growing from their challenges.

A Biblical Step 12

☑ Allow God's love to flow through you to others; the more we give, the more we receive.

Science has revealed that even though we may avoid unhealthy behaviors (taking a substance, gambling, shopping) if we engage in the behavior in our imagination, the same neural circuits fire as when the actual behavior is carried out.

The Bible Says...

We don't use worldly weapons designed to kill the body or destroy physical structures, nor do we use the world's weapons of lies, distortion, manipulation, deceit, flattery, coercion, sanctions, or trickery. On the contrary, our weapons are from God and have divine power to free the mind, heal the heart, and demolish Satan's stronghold of fear, lies and selfishness. We demolish every idea, argument, doctrine, teaching or concept that infects the mind and distorts or obstructs the truth about God, and we reclaim the thoughts, feelings and attitudes into the truth about God as revealed by Jesus Christ. We stand ready to bring discipline to bear to help break destructive habits so that maturity and health will be fully realized.
(2 Corinthians 10:4-6 REM)

CHAPTER 17

AVOIDANCE & DEFENSIVE BEHAVIOR

Breaking Free from the Shackles of Avoidance & Defense Behavior with Biblical Wisdom and Inspiring Guidance

When it comes to addiction recovery, many individuals, even those of Christian faith, struggle with avoidance and defense behavior, which can lead to relapse. Avoiding triggers and engaging in defense mechanisms may seem like a means of self-preservation, but they often hinder the healing process. As genuine followers of Christ Jesus, the renewal of heart and mind compels us to face our struggles head-on, seeking the strength and guidance of our Lord. Through His transformative power, we can truly break free from the grips of addiction. We can find lasting recovery by confronting the underlying issues and replacing avoidance and defense mechanisms with healthy coping mechanisms. Philippians 4:13 (AMP) says, *"I can do all things [which He has called me to do] through Him who strengthens and empowers me [to fulfill His purpose—I am self-sufficient in Christ's sufficiency; I am ready for anything and equal to anything through Him who infuses me with inner strength and confident peace.]"* As we journey towards freedom from addiction, let us hold on to this verse, drawing inspiration from it.

In addiction relapse, various factors contribute to individuals' prevalent avoidance and defense behaviors. One primary cause lies in the *Faulty Beliefs* ingrained within their minds. These distorted perceptions often stem from deep-seated *Fears*, perpetuating a cycle of *Defensiveness* and *Contrariness*. Moreover, *Impulsiveness* plays a significant role as it leads to impulsive decision-making, furthering the path toward relapse. Another contributing factor is *Loneliness*, as individuals may seek comfort in addictive substances or behaviors to escape for self-soothing.

Nevertheless, it is vital to remember that through faith guidance, individuals can find the strength to overcome these challenges. Seeking inspiration from biblical references can offer clarity and motivation to combat addiction. By fostering a belief in oneself and the power of transformation, individuals can break free from addiction and embark on a journey toward healing and restoration.

Avoidance & Defense Characteristics

1. Faulty Beliefs:

Faulty beliefs trigger addiction relapse because they undermine the very foundation of recovery. In the battle against addiction, our thoughts and ideas are pivotal in determining our success or failure. As a Christian, it is crucial to understand the spiritual implications of addiction and how our beliefs can either empower or hinder our journey toward healing and wholeness.

Addiction is a complex and multifaceted issue, encompassing physical, psychological, and spiritual dimensions. In recovery, many often overlook the spiritual component, while detoxification and therapy address the physical and psychological aspects. Faulty beliefs can manifest in various ways, such as doubting God's healing ability, feeling unworthy of forgiveness, or believing that addiction defines one's identity.

To truly overcome addiction, it is crucial to align our beliefs with the truth found in the Bible. The Word of God offers a powerful source of strength, wisdom, and hope. It reminds us that we are fearfully and wonderfully made (Psalm 139:14) and that with God, all things are possible (Matthew 19:26). By embracing these truths, we can counter the faulty beliefs that trigger relapse and cultivate a mindset of victory and transformation.

One faulty belief that often leads to relapse is that addiction is a lifelong sentence, an impossible burden. However, the Bible teaches us that in Christ, we are new creations (2 Corinthians 5:17) and that through Him, we can do all things (Philippians 4:13). By internalizing these truths, we can replace the belief in an endless struggle with the trust in God's redemptive power to break the chains of addiction.

Another faulty belief triggering relapse is self-reliance. Many individuals struggling with addiction fall into the trap of thinking they can overcome their dependency. This self-sufficiency mindset often leads to isolation and a lack of accountability, making relapse more likely. The Bible, however, emphasizes the importance of community and support. Proverbs 27:17 (AMP) reminds us that *"As iron sharpens iron, So one man sharpens [and influences] another [through discussion]."* This highlights the need for companionship and mutual encouragement. We need accountability and support. By embracing this truth, individuals can seek help from fellow believers, accountability partners, and support groups, strengthening their recovery journey.

Faulty beliefs also affect our understanding of forgiveness and grace. Many individuals feel unworthy of God's forgiveness, leading to self-condemnation and hopelessness.

However, Romans 8:1-4 (REM) assures us, *"Therefore, those who trust in Christ Jesus are no longer destined to die, because through Christ Jesus the law of love has cleansed and healed them from the law of selfishness and death. The written law was powerless to restore trust, as it could merely diagnose the infection of distrust and selfishness pervading us all. God accomplished this restoration of his character of love in humans by sending his own Son in human flesh to eradicate selfishness from humanity, reveal the truth about God, expose the lies of Satan, and reveal what happens when the infection of sin is not cured. And so he condemned the infection of selfishness as the destroying element in sinful humanity in order that the law of love—the principle upon which life is based—might be fully restored in us, who no longer live according to selfish desires, but in harmony with the Spirit of love and truth.*"

This powerful verse reminds us that God's forgiveness is unconditional and limitless. No matter how grave our mistakes may be, God's grace is always available to us.

"*Those who live with the selfish nature in charge [active addictive personality] have their minds bent on selfindulgence and selfish pursuits; but those who live in harmony with the Spirit of truth and love have their minds focused on living in harmony with God's principles of truth, love, and liberty.*" (Romans 8:5 REM; emphasis mine)

Yet, faulty beliefs can cloud our understanding of this profound truth. We may falsely believe that we need to earn God's forgiveness or that our sins are too great to be forgiven. These misconceptions can weigh heavily on our hearts, causing us to doubt God's love and mercy.

The Bible is evident in its teachings about forgiveness and grace. Ephesians 2:8-10 (REM) affirms, "*It is only because of God's grace that you have been healed through trust—and you did not create this trust yourself, but it was established through the evidence of God's character revealed in the gift of Jesus Christ. This is not by some human work—No way!—so there is no room for anyone to boast. We are God's special creation brought to existence by Christ Jesus to showcase his character—his living law of love—which was always God's design for us.*" God's abundant grace is the precursor to our salvation and forgiveness, not our efforts or worthiness. —see Galatians 3

Understanding this truth can bring immense freedom and healing to our lives. When we realize that God's forgiveness is not dependent on our actions or past mistakes, we can let go of the burden of guilt and shame. We can embrace the transformative power of God's grace and allow it to shape our lives.

Furthermore, faulty beliefs about forgiveness can hinder our ability to extend grace to others. If we struggle to accept God's forgiveness for ourselves, we may find it difficult to forgive others. We may hold onto grudges and resentments, allowing bitterness to poison our relationships.

However, as followers of Christ, we are called to emulate His example of forgiveness. In Matthew 6:14-15 (REM), Jesus teaches us,

"For it is when you forgive others their wrongs that your heart is open to receive the forgiving and healing power your heavenly Father extends to you. But if you harden your heart and refuse to forgive others their sins, your heart is closed and unable to receive the forgiveness your heavenly Father extends to you." This powerful reminder urges us to let go of our grievances and forgive those who wronged us.

When we embrace the truth of God's forgiveness and extend grace to others, we experience the transformative power of love and reconciliation. We release ourselves from resentment and bitterness, allowing healing and restoration.

Faulty beliefs about forgiveness and grace can hinder our understanding and experience of God's unconditional love. However, the Bible offers clear guidance, assuring us that God's forgiveness is limitless and His grace is freely given. By embracing this truth, we can find freedom from self-condemnation, cultivate healthy relationships, and experience the transformative power of God's love. Hold firm to these truths, allowing them to shape our perspective and guide our actions. As we strive to live out God's love in our lives, let us remember that forgiveness and grace are not merely concepts to be understood intellectually but truths embraced wholeheartedly.

In Ephesians 4:32 (REM), the apostle Paul reminds us to *"Be kind, gentle, compassionate and forgiving with each other as God is forgiving to you; remember that all humanity suffers with the same infection of selfishness, and God provides the same Remedy for all."* This verse serves as a potent reminder that our forgiveness of others is rooted in our forgiveness of God. It is a reflection of His grace and mercy towards us.

Moreover, the Bible assures us that God's forgiveness knows no limits. In Psalm 103:12 (NIV), we read, *"As far as the East is from the West, so far has he removed our transgressions from us."* This beautiful imagery emphasizes the boundless nature of God's forgiveness. When we confess our sins and seek His forgiveness, He forgives us and removes our sins from us entirely.

Embracing forgiveness and grace allows us to cultivate healthy relationships with others. When we recognize the forgiveness we have received from God, it becomes easier for us to extend that same forgiveness to those who have wronged us. As Jesus taught in 2 Corinthians 2:5-8 (NIV), *"If anyone has caused grief, he has not so much grieved me as he has grieved all of you to some extent—not to put it too severely. The punishment inflicted on him by the majority is sufficient. Now instead, you ought to forgive and comfort him, so that he will not be overwhelmed by excessive sorrow. I urge you therefore, to reaffirm your love for him."* By choosing to forgive, we honor God's command and create an atmosphere of reconciliation and restoration in our relationships.

Finally, embracing forgiveness and grace opens the door to experiencing the transformative power of God's love. When we allow His forgiveness to wash over us, we are freed from the burdens of the past and empowered to live a life of purpose and fulfillment. God's grace enables us to live out our true identity as beloved children of God, capable of great love and compassion for others —Forgiving takes the monkey off your back.

2. Fears:

Fear triggers addiction relapse because it taps into our deepest vulnerabilities and unsettles our sense of security. Addiction often arises as a coping mechanism to escape anxiety, pain, or trauma. When faced with fear-inducing situations, individuals may turn to substances or behaviors that provide temporary relief or distraction. However, this detrimental cycle perpetuates the addiction, as the quick escape ultimately increases the fear and anxiety in the long run.

The Bible provides guidance and wisdom on overcoming fear and addiction. 2 Timothy 1:7 (REM) states, *"For God did not give you a character of insecurity, doubt, and fear, but a mind and character of confidence, power in the truth, love, and self-control."* This verse reminds us that fear does not come from God but rather from the enemy who seeks to rob us of our peace and joy. It encourages us to rely on God's power, love, and soundness of mind to overcome fear and addiction.

A lack of healthy coping mechanisms also triggers addiction relapse. When individuals face fearful situations, they may resort to their addictive behaviors as a means to regain control or numb their emotions. Developing alternative strategies and tools to manage fear and anxiety is essential. The Bible provides numerous examples of seeking God's guidance, prayer, and solace in His promises. By turning to God and His word, we can find strength, peace, and comfort in times of fear and uncertainty.

Moreover, a distorted perception that substances or behaviors can alleviate fear often drives addiction relapse. This mindset stems from the false belief that addiction solves life's challenges. However, addiction only exacerbates the underlying problems, leading to a vicious cycle of dependency and fear. Recognizing this fallacy is crucial to breaking free from addiction and finding true healing.

Overcoming fear and addiction requires a holistic approach that addresses our life's physical, emotional, and spiritual aspects. Seeking professional help, such as counseling or therapy, can provide valuable insights and support. Additionally, connecting with a supportive community, such as a church or recovery group, can offer encouragement and accountability.

Ultimately, finding freedom from addiction and fear requires deep faith in God's power to transform lives. The Bible, considered by Christians as the ultimate authority, offers guidance and reassurance in overcoming these struggles. In Isaiah 41:10 (NIV), a verse frequently quoted for its profound impact, God speaks directly to His people, saying, "*So do not fear, for I am with you; do not be dismayed, for I am your God. I will strengthen you and help you; I will uphold you with my righteous right hand.*"

These words from the book of Isaiah hold significant weight and offer hope to those grappling with addiction and fear. They remind us that we are not alone in our battles. God's presence is a constant source of strength and comfort. With unwavering faith, we can trust that He will guide us through the darkest times, empowering us to conquer our addictions and fears.

The transformative power of God's love is beautifully exemplified throughout the Bible. Countless stories highlight individuals once bound by addiction finding liberation and healing through their trust in God. For instance, the prodigal son's story illustrates God's unconditional love and forgiveness, showing that His mercy is always available no matter how far we have strayed.

It is essential to understand that overcoming addiction and fear is a process that requires perseverance and dedication. It may involve seeking professional help, joining support groups, or engaging in therapy. However, the foundation of lasting transformation lies in developing an unshakable faith in God's power and ability to restore and renew.

By immersing ourselves in the teachings of the Bible, we gain invaluable wisdom and guidance. The scriptures provide a roadmap for living free from addiction and fear. They offer practical principles, such as self-control, perseverance, and reliance on God's strength. We find peace, clarity, and the motivation to press on through prayer and meditation on God's word.

In our journey toward freedom, we must surround ourselves with a community of like-minded believers who can provide encouragement, support, and accountability. Together, we can share our struggles, offer insights, and uplift one another in prayer. The strength of a united community rooted in faith is a powerful force in overcoming addiction and fear.

As we walk this path toward freedom, we must remember that setbacks and challenges are inevitable. However, God's promise in Isaiah 41:10 remains steadfast. He assures us that He will strengthen and uphold us, guiding us through the storms of life.

In our journey toward freedom, anchoring ourselves in God's words is crucial. His wisdom and guidance provide us with the strength and courage to overcome any obstacle that may come our way. The Bible is a timeless source of inspiration and motivation, offering clarity and insight into our path.

Reflecting on the words of Isaiah 41:10, we find serenity in the knowledge that God is always by our side. He promises to strengthen us physically, emotionally, and spiritually. In times of weakness and doubt, His unwavering support sustains us and gives us the energy to persevere.

Moreover, when we face challenges on our path toward freedom, we can find comfort in the assurance that God will uphold us. He will lift and prevent us from stumbling, ensuring our steps remain secure and steadfast. With God as our guide, we can navigate the treacherous terrain of life with confidence and determination.

I do not believe it is God's intention for us to be discouraged by setbacks and challenges. Instead, I see them as opportunities for growth and transformation. As we face these obstacles head-on, we develop resilience and deepen our faith. Amid adversity, God's presence strengthens us, allowing us to rise above our circumstances and reach new heights.

In our pursuit of freedom, let us hold onto the promises found in Isaiah 41:10. Let us trust in God's unwavering love and guidance, knowing He will provide us with the strength we need. As we face setbacks and challenges, let us be reminded of His words and draw inspiration from the wisdom of the Bible.

May the assurance of God's presence and His promise to strengthen and uphold us guide our journey toward liberty. With faith as our compass and the Bible as our source of inspiration, we can navigate life's uncertainties with clarity and determination. Let us embrace the challenges that come our way, for they are stepping stones toward true freedom.

3. Defensiveness:

Defensiveness triggers addiction relapse because it hinders the essential process of self-reflection and growth. Addiction recovery is a delicate journey that requires individuals to confront their past, address underlying issues, and make positive life changes. However, defensiveness can be a significant obstacle, preventing individuals from fully engaging in this transformative process.

When individuals become defensive, they erect emotional barriers that shield them from acknowledging their mistakes, weaknesses, and vulnerabilities. Instead of taking responsibility for their actions, they shift the blame onto others or external circumstances. This defensive stance perpetuates a cycle of denial and avoidance, hindering the necessary steps toward lasting recovery.

Moreover, defensiveness fosters a mindset of resistance to change. Addiction recovery necessitates a willingness to explore uncomfortable emotions, face the consequences of past behaviors, and embrace personal growth. However, when individuals are defensive, they resist this change, clinging to old behavior and thought patterns. This resistance acts as a gravitational force, pulling them back into the familiar territory of addiction.

The Bible emphasizes the importance of humility and self-reflection in Christian teachings. Proverbs 28:13 (NIV) states, *"Whoever conceals their sins does not prosper, but the one who confesses and renounces them finds mercy."* This verse encourages individuals to confront their wrongdoings and seek forgiveness from God and themselves. By embracing humility and acknowledging their vulnerabilities, individuals can break free from addiction and find the strength to rebuild their lives.

To overcome defensiveness and prevent addiction relapse, individuals must cultivate a mindset of self-awareness and openness. To do so involves:

- Acknowledging their mistakes.
- Accepting feedback from loved ones and professionals.
- Seeking guidance and support from a community of like-minded individuals.

By engaging in regular self-reflection, individuals can identify their triggers, recognize patterns of defensiveness, and work towards healthier coping mechanisms.

Furthermore, it is crucial to develop practical communication skills. Learning to express emotions and concerns constructively can help individuals address conflicts and challenges without resorting to defensiveness. Building healthy relationships and establishing a support network of individuals who understand the struggles of addiction recovery can provide the necessary encouragement and accountability to stay on track.

Defensiveness acts as a stumbling block on the path to addiction recovery. By acknowledging our vulnerabilities, embracing humility, and fostering self-awareness, we can break free from the cycle of defensiveness and find the strength to overcome addiction. Let us draw inspiration from the teachings of the Bible and remember that true freedom and transformation lie in our ability to let go of defensiveness and surrender to a higher power. As the book of Proverbs states, *"Pride leads to destruction, and arrogance to downfall."* (Proverbs 16:18 GNT)

Defensiveness often stems from a fear of judgment or a desire to protect our egos. However, in the journey toward addiction recovery, it is crucial to confront these fears head-on and allow ourselves to be vulnerable. Doing so opens the doors to self-reflection, growth, and healing.

Embracing humility is a powerful tool on this path. It allows us to recognize our limitations and acknowledge that we cannot overcome addiction alone. We must be willing to seek support from others, whether it be through counseling, support groups, or the guidance of a higher power. In the words of James 4:5-6 (REM), *"Don't you get it? The Scripture is clear: God longs intensely for you and gives his Spirit to live in you to graciously heal you. That is why the Scripture says: 'God opposes selfishness, arrogance and pride, but heals the selfless.'"*

Self-awareness is another crucial aspect of breaking free from defensiveness. By examining our thoughts, emotions, and behaviors with honesty and clarity, we can identify the underlying causes of our addiction and make necessary changes. The Bible encourages self-examination. Psalm 139:23-24 (REM) states, "Examine me, O God, and know the deepest recesses of my heart; test me and identify every troublesome thought. Determine if there is any unhealthy way in me, and lead me back to everlasting life."

In this process, it is essential to remember that addiction recovery is not a linear journey. There may be setbacks and challenges, but we can find the strength to persevere by surrendering our defensiveness. The Apostle Paul writes in James 1:2-4 (REM), *"My brothers and sisters in God's family, I want you to rejoice and keep a positive attitude whenever you face troubles of various kinds, because every trial exercises your trust in God–which overcomes fear and selfishness–and builds a confident, steadfast application of the Remedy. And this steadfast engagement in God's treatment must be completed so that you may be fully healed, mature, and like Christ in character–not lacking anything."*

Letting go of defensiveness opens us to true freedom and transformation. The Bible provides wisdom and guidance in this pursuit, reminding us of the importance of humility, self-awareness, and reliance on a higher power. Remember these teachings as we navigate the path to addiction recovery, knowing we can find the strength to overcome with God's grace and willingness to surrender.

4. Contrariness:

Contrariness triggers addiction relapse because it tempts individuals to stray from their path of recovery. Addiction is a complex and multifaceted issue requiring unwavering commitment and dedication. However, when confronted with contrary thoughts, beliefs, or circumstances, individuals may find themselves at a crossroads where the temptation to revert to their addictive behaviors becomes overwhelming.

In the pursuit of recovery, it is crucial to understand the power of contrariness. It can manifest in various forms, such as never-ending doubts, skepticism, or even external pressures from those who do not fully grasp the challenges of addiction. Can it be called defiance and opposition? These contrary influences can shake the foundations of one's resolve, leading to a relapse.

1. James 4:7 — *"Submit yourselves, then, to God. Resist the devil, and he will flee from you."* This verse emphasizes the importance of submitting to God's will and resisting external temptations or adversarial forces, which can be akin to the opposition faced in recovery.

2. Ephesians 6:13 — *"Therefore put on the full armor of God, so that when the day of evil comes, you may be able to stand your ground, and after you have done everything, to stand."* This

passage speaks to being prepared for times of challenge (the 'day of evil') and equipping oneself spiritually to withstand and overcome contrary influences.

3. 1 Peter 5:8-9 — *"Be alert and of sober mind. Your enemy the devil prowls around like a roaring lion looking for someone to devour. Resist him, standing firm in the faith, because you know that the family of believers throughout the world is undergoing the same kind of sufferings."* Here, the call to be vigilant and resist opposition is clear. It also connects individual struggles with those of a wider community, offering a sense of solidarity and commonality in facing adversities.

4. Romans 12:21 — *"Do not be overcome by evil, but overcome evil with good."* This verse can be particularly motivational in recovery, suggesting that one can counter negative influences (or contrariness) by resisting and actively pursuing good.

In standing firm with recovery, it is imperative to fortify oneself with the necessary tools and mindset. Drawing inspiration from the Bible, we find numerous examples of individuals who overcame adversity through unwavering faith and determination. Their stories serve as beacons of hope and encouragement, reminding us that we, too, can conquer the trials that come our way.

Moreover, seeking support from a strong faith community can provide the necessary guidance and motivation to navigate the treacherous waters of addiction recovery. Surrounding oneself with individuals who understand the struggles and can offer wise counsel can be instrumental in resisting the allure of contrary influences.

Additionally, it is essential to maintain clarity of purpose and remind ourselves why we embarked on the journey of recovery in the first place. Reflecting on the detrimental effects of addiction on our physical, mental, and spiritual well-being can serve as a powerful deterrent against relapse. Keeping our goals and aspirations at the forefront of our minds strengthens our resolve and remains steadfast even in the face of contrariness.

Ultimately, the battle against addiction requires a holistic approach that combines faith, knowledge, and unwavering determination. By recognizing the potential triggers of relapse, such as contrariness, we can equip ourselves with the necessary tools and strategies to overcome them. Let us draw inspiration from the Bible, seek support from our faith community, and remain focused on our ultimate goal of freedom from addiction. With God's grace and our unwavering commitment, we can conquer contrariness and embrace a life of lasting recovery and fulfillment.

5. Impulsiveness:

Impulsiveness triggers addiction relapse because it allows individuals to surrender to their immediate desires, disregarding the long-term consequences that addiction brings. Addiction is a complex and insidious condition that affects millions of lives worldwide. It exerts a powerful hold over individuals, making breaking free from its grasp difficult. However, understanding the role of impulsiveness in addiction relapse can provide valuable insights into the recovery process.

The Bible emphasizes self-control as a virtue that helps individuals resist temptation and make wise choices. Proverbs 25:28 (AMP) states, *"Like a city that is broken down and without walls [leaving it unprotected] Is a man who has no self-control over his spirit [and sets himself up for trouble]."* Impulsiveness, on the other hand, can be likened to a breach in these walls, allowing the destructive forces of addiction to infiltrate and take control once again.

Addiction relapse often occurs when individuals succumb to impulsive behavior, failing to resist the allure of their addictive substance or behavior. Addiction's immediate gratification can overpower rational thinking and cloud one's judgment. This lack of self-control can lead to a downward spiral, reigniting the cycle of addiction and jeopardizing the progress made in recovery. Control what you think to control what you do.

It is crucial to recognize that addiction is not solely a physical dependence but also a psychological and spiritual struggle. By addressing the underlying issues that fuel impulsive behavior, individuals can better understand their addiction and develop the necessary tools to overcome it.

Motivation plays a pivotal role in recovery, and individuals must find a vital source of inspiration to counter their impulsive tendencies. Connecting with their faith and seeking guidance from God can provide the clarity and strength needed to resist temptation. James 4:7 (REM) advises, *"Surrender yourselves to God and his treatment. Tell the devil No, and you will escape him. 8 Move close to God, and God will come close to you. You selfish people! Stop choosing to indulge your desires. Stop going back and forth between love and selfishness, and purify your hearts with love."* Individuals can find the motivation and strength to break free from addiction by surrendering their impulsive desires to a higher power, God.

Recovery is a journey that requires perseverance and a commitment to personal growth. Effective strategies to manage impulsivity, such as counseling, support groups, and practical coping mechanisms, are essential. By consciously practicing self-control and making deliberate choices, individuals can gradually regain control over their lives and reduce the risk of addiction relapse.

Impulsiveness can act as a catalyst for addiction relapse, as it undermines self-control and impairs sound judgment. However, by comprehending the role of impulsivity in addiction, individuals can gain the necessary knowledge to develop effective strategies for resisting temptation and making healthier choices. Seeking guidance from biblical principles and relying on the teachings of our Christian faith can provide invaluable insight and motivation in this journey toward recovery.

The Bible offers timeless wisdom and practical advice that can help individuals overcome impulsive behavior and break free from the chains of addiction. Proverbs 16:32 reminds us, *"Whoever is slow to anger is better than the mighty, and he who rules his spirit than he who takes a city."* This verse emphasizes the importance of self-control in all aspects of our lives, including overcoming addiction.

Additionally, the Apostle Paul provides guidance in Galatians 5:22-23, where he speaks of the fruits of the Spirit, one of which is self-control. By allowing the Holy Spirit to work within us, we can find the strength to resist impulsive urges and make choices that align with our desire for a healthier and more fulfilling life.

Also, the Bible instructs us to renew our minds and transform our thinking. Romans 12:2 (REM) encourages us, *"Do not continue to practice the destructive methods of selfishness, which infect the world, but be completely transformed into God's image by the renewing of your mind. Then you will value God's principles, practice his methods, and discern his will—his good, pleasing, and perfect will."* By renewing our minds with God's Word, we can gain clarity and discernment, making it easier to resist impulsive behaviors and make choices that honor our commitment to sobriety.

In addition to seeking guidance from biblical principles, it is crucial to surround ourselves with a supportive community of fellow believers. Hebrews 10:24-25 (NIV) states, *"And let us consider how to stir up one another to love and good works, not neglecting to meet together, as is the habit of some, but encouraging one another, and all the more as you see the Day drawing near."* This passage emphasizes the importance of gathering together to encourage and motivate each other, which is crucial in a recovery context. By connecting with like-minded individuals who share our faith and are committed to living a life free from addiction, we can find encouragement, accountability, and inspiration to stay on the path of recovery.

Ultimately, understanding the role of impulsivity in addiction and incorporating biblical principles into our recovery journey empowers us to make positive strides toward a healthier and more fulfilling life. By relying on God's guidance, we can find the strength to resist temptation, exercise self-control, and make choices that align with our desire for lasting sobriety. Let us be inspired by the teachings of our Christian faith and motivated by the promise of a renewed life in Christ.

6. Loneliness:

Loneliness triggers addiction relapse because it preys upon the vulnerable and unsettled hearts of individuals whom the weight of addiction has already burdened. During these moments of isolation, the allure of substance abuse becomes more enticing, as it promises temporary relief from the pain of loneliness.

In the Bible, we see numerous examples of individuals who faced loneliness and its profound impact on their lives; for instance, King David was tempted to succumb to his desires in his moments of solitude. During one of these moments, he fell into the trap of lust and committed adultery with Bathsheba (2 Samuel 11:1-4). David's loneliness allowed the darkness within him to overpower his sense of righteousness, leading him down a destructive path.

Loneliness can also be seen as a breeding ground for negative thoughts and emotions, creating a void many seek to fill with addictive substances. It is during these times that individuals may turn to drugs, alcohol, or other vices in an attempt to escape their feelings of isolation. The addictive nature of these substances only further perpetuates the cycle of loneliness, as they provide a temporary escape but ultimately deepen the sense of isolation and despair.

However, it is crucial to remember that there is hope beyond the grip of addiction and loneliness. The Bible offers us guidance and encouragement to overcome these challenges. Psalm 34:17-20 (REM) states, "*Those set right with God call to him and he answers them; he heals them from all their sin-sickness. The Lord stays close to the grief-stricken and heartbroken and heals those who humbly allow him to. Those whose hearts are right with God may have many problems in life, but the Lord saves despite life's troubles; he watches over his faithful — keeping them strong like bones —they will not be broken.*" These words remind us that God is with us even in our deepest despair, offering comfort and strength.

It is vital to seek support from a community of like-minded individuals who can provide encouragement, accountability, and love to overcome addiction and its loneliness. Surrounding oneself with positive influences and engaging in healthy activities can help fill the void left by addiction. Developing a solid spiritual foundation through prayer, Biblical meditation, and reading the Bible can provide guidance and a sense of purpose.

Loneliness may trigger addiction relapse, but it does not have to define our lives. Through trust in God, perseverance, and the support of others, we can overcome the darkness that seeks to consume us. Let us draw strength from the teachings of the Bible, find solace in the presence of God, and embrace the journey toward healing and freedom from addiction.

When embarking on the journey of addiction recovery, it is crucial for individuals, including those with Christian faith, to recognize the pitfalls of avoidance and defense behavior. While it may initially appear to be a means of self-protection, these actions can ultimately impede the healing process and pave the way for relapse. As genuine followers of Christ Jesus, it is crucial to face our struggles head-on, forsaking the crutches of triggers and defense mechanisms. Instead, we should anchor our hearts and minds in Him, seeking His strength and guidance to navigate the path to freedom. We can break free from addiction through His transformative power and find proper restoration. So let us let go of avoidance and defense and embrace the transformative journey that lies ahead, empowered by our faith and the steadfast love of our Lord.

The Bible Says...

Those set right with God call to HIM and HE answers them; HE heals them from all their sin-sickness. The LORD stays close to the grief-stricken and heartbroken and heals those who humbly allow HIM to. Those whose hearts are right with God may have many problems in life, but the LORD saves despite life's troubles; HE watches over HIS faithful — keeping them strong like bones —they will not be broken. (Psalm 34:17-20, REM)

CHAPTER 18

CRISIS BUILDING

Turning Point or Critical Hurdle: The Dual Nature of Crisis Building in Addiction Recovery

Crisis building refers to a process within addiction recovery where an individual or their support network may consciously or unconsciously amplify a situation to bring about a realization, intervention, or decisive change. However, the difference can be positive or negative depending upon the choices of the one in recovery. It can be both a turning point and a critical hurdle in the recovery process.

Crisis building can occur at any stage of recovery, but it's prevalent during the contemplation, action, and maintenance stages. This is a crucial point to remember as we navigate the challenges of personal growth and transformation. In times of crisis, we often question our abilities, feel overwhelmed, and doubt whether we have what it takes to overcome obstacles.

As Christians, we can find comfort and guidance in the words of the Bible. In times of crisis, it is crucial to turn to the bible passages for inspiration and clarity. One verse that resonates with this topic is in 2 Corinthians 12:9 (NIV), where it says, *"But he said to me, 'My grace is sufficient for you, for my power is made perfect in weakness.' Therefore, I will boast all the more gladly about my weaknesses so that Christ's power may rest on me."*

This verse reminds us that in moments of crisis, when we feel weak and inadequate, God's grace is more than enough to sustain us. His power can shine through our weaknesses, giving us the strength and resilience to overcome any obstacles.

Furthermore, the Bible teaches us that crisis building can be an opportunity for growth and transformation. Romans 5:3-5 (REM) states, *"Because of this, we rejoice in our trials and afflictions, for we know that trials bring to light our shortcomings and defects of character. If we persevere, choosing God's methods, the defects are removed and character is purified, and pure character increases our hope for God's kingdom. And our hope will not be disappointed, because God pours out his love into our hearts and thereby matures, ennobles, and restores us into his image by the Holy Spirit, whom he has given to us."* This passage reminds us that through the challenges and crises we encounter, we can develop perseverance, which builds character and ultimately leads to hope.

Staying motivated and focused on our goals is crucial as we navigate the contemplation, action, and maintenance stages of recovery. Surrounding ourselves with like-minded individuals who can offer support and encouragement can be helpful. Additionally, seeking guidance from trusted mentors or spiritual leaders can provide us with valuable insights and perspectives to navigate through the crisis-building process.

Crisis building is not meant to break us but to mold us into stronger individuals. In times of crisis, we can tap into our inner strength and rely on the power of God's grace. By embracing our weaknesses and seeking guidance from the scriptures during the entirety of recovery, we can find the inspiration and motivation to persevere through any challenges that come our way.

Let no crisis be wasted! Let's find ways to use a crisis to drive us closer to God and be encouraged and inspired by the words of the Bible as we navigate the stages of recovery.

To enhance one's abilities, the primary objective of this section is to reduce the occurrence of unfavorable choices when faced with challenging situations. During recovery, the intense pressure associated with crisis building often leads to various difficulties. These challenges include *self-destructive behavior, feelings of entitlement, division within oneself, insufficient preparation, rigid thinking, and feelings of depression.*

Self-Destructive Behavior

The trouble with self-destructive behavior, also known as self-sabotaging during addiction recovery, hinders the progress and growth one needs to overcome their struggles.

During recovery, when someone engages in self-sabotage, there is a conflict between how they perceive themselves and how others perceive them. This conflict arises from the pressure to meet the expectations and opinions of others, as well as a weakened self-image where they may feel inferior, constantly seek validation, or believe they are not capable enough. Self-defeating behavior undermines their self-worth, dignity, and sense of identity, consequently affecting their relationships, which is not desirable.

To address and change this behavior during recovery, it is essential first to identify the triggers or underlying issues causing it. Identifying triggers involves:

- Engaging in honest self-reflection
- Being open to change
- Having a solid determination to follow through despite the challenges that may arise

While some individuals can make these changes independently, it can also be beneficial to have the support and accountability of caring and reliable friends and family.

The temptations to revert to old habits or fall into destructive patterns can be overwhelming, but it is vital to remember the teachings of the Bible and draw strength from it. Scripture reminds us that we are called to renew our minds and not conform to the patterns of this world (Romans 12:2).

With God's guidance, we can overcome self-sabotaging by following three steps:

1. Learn what is morally correct by immersing yourself in studying God's Word.
2. Cultivate a genuine desire to align our hearts and desires with the Holy Spirit's guidance, asking for His transformative intervention.
3. Implement righteous actions that maintain our commitment to doing what is right.

By adhering to these principles, we find the strength and motivation to combat self-sabotage effectively, ultimately leading to personal growth and fulfillment in our Christian journey.

When allowing ourselves to be vulnerable to sabotage, we risk delaying the transformation we desperately seek. Instead, adhere to the promise of redemption and the power of God's grace to guide us toward a life free from addiction. Through prayer, support systems, and personal vigilance, we can overcome the allure of self-sabotage and embrace the blessings of a sobriety-lived life. Even during a struggle, God's grace is always sufficient (2 Corinthians 12:9). So, have faith, persevere, and stay on the path to recovery, for it is a journey filled with hope and endless possibilities.

Feelings of Entitlement

Entitlement is the belief that one inherently deserves privileges or special treatment. In addiction recovery, this attitude may manifest in various ways, including a lack of personal responsibility associated with pride, unrealistic expectations, and resistance to change.

Beliefs of entitlement may stem from a person's mental or emotional state or socio-cultural factors, such as narcissistic personality traits, overindulgence in childhood, or a cultural emphasis on individual rights and freedoms.

An entitlement mentality often includes a belief that external factors rather than personal choices cause one's problems. In addiction recovery, this may lead to blaming others or circumstances for addictive behavior rather than recognizing personal responsibility for change.

Entitlement can also foster unrealistic expectations about the recovery process. Individuals may expect instant success without effort or believe they deserve special treatment in their recovery program. Expectations of privilege can lead to disappointment and frustration, undermining motivation and commitment.

A person with an entitled mindset may resist making necessary changes in behavior, lifestyle, or thinking patterns, believing they don't need to conform to typical recovery protocols. This resistance can hinder progress and potentially lead to relapse.

From a Christian perspective, the trouble with entitlement during addiction recovery is pride. Entitlement contrasts the virtues of humility and self-sacrifice, which are essential for personal transformation and growth. Surrendering to God as a higher power and accepting one's limitations aligns with the values that often facilitate a successful recovery.

The Bible identifies the entitled by saying, *"Their pride and arrogance are flaunted like a necklace; violence and exploitation cover them."* (Psalm 73:6 REM) Recovery requires humility, surrender, and a deep reliance on a higher power.

Entitlement, however, is rooted in self-centeredness—egocentricity—and instant gratification, hindering individuals from embracing the necessary compliance for lasting recovery.

True transformation requires a humble heart, recognizing one's limitations, and being willing to submit to God's guidance. In recovery, this means setting aside our entitlement by acknowledging the need for God's grace and counsel with a spirit of gratitude, perseverance, and selflessness.

The Apostle Paul presents a powerful reminder that Christ willingly relinquished his rights (entitlements) so that we could partake in his magnificence (Philippians 2:5–8). As believers, our trust in God should extend beyond moments of unmet desires. Inspired by the selflessness of our Savior, please let go of perceived entitlements willingly. By following this divine example, we can find inspiration and clarity in our Christian journey through genuine addiction recovery.

Division Within Oneself

In addiction recovery, the emergence of internal division, such as splitting, presents a formidable obstacle. This defense mechanism also called black-and-white thinking, involves perceiving oneself and others solely in terms of good or bad, devoid of any middle ground. Splitting poses a significant challenge and requires a profound understanding of the cognitive processes involved.

An example of splitting involves directing one's romantic partner to depart and pleading with them to stay once they have left. A shared spoken theme is "I hate you...Don't leave me!" In addition, it entails assigning another person's actions solely to their inherent righteousness or wickedness rather than recognizing them as multifaceted individuals with a combination of positive, negative, and neutral qualities.

In addiction recovery, division within oneself or splitting defense mechanisms can be detrimental, hindering self-reflection, growth, and the ability to establish meaningful connections. By dividing the self (or others) into either entirely good or entirely bad entities, individuals with addiction tendencies fail to acknowledge their complexities or accept their mistakes. Therefore, those in recovery must recognize the limitations of splitting and embrace a more balanced perspective.

Splitting creates a barrier to growth and impedes the formation of a healthy self-image. The journey towards recovery requires a compassionate perspective and a willingness to confront the truth within ourselves. In doing so, we can unlock the transformative power of self-love and regain control of our lives. By acknowledging and working through the challenges associated with this defense mechanism, individuals can foster personal growth, cultivate healthy relationships, and find the strength to overcome addiction.

Within the teachings of the Bible, we find guidance and wisdom to overcome this challenge. As believers, we are issued the entire armor of God. This armor equips our minds with all the necessary tools to join the ranks of Christ's soldiers and confidently withstand the devil's schemes. It is essential, therefore, to fortify our minds with God's complete set of spiritual armor. The Spirit-issued protective covering will enable us to stand firm, even in the face of Satan's grand deception, when it feels as though the very foundations of heaven are shaking. We must remain steadfast and unwavering, even when tempted to falter. Let us stand firm, always presenting the truth and exposing Satan's lies (Ephesians 6:11, 13).

Insufficient Preparation

Insufficient planning in addiction recovery can lead to a crisis in various ways, creating obstacles for the individual and the professionals involved in their care. The trouble with insufficient preparation or poor planning during addiction recovery is that it can hinder progress and perpetuate cycles of relapse.

A few of the underlying causes of insufficient preparation leading to relapse:

- The lack of understanding of addiction as a disease rather than a moral failing can lead to insufficient planning.
- Resource constraints within lifestyle or treatment facilities, such as inadequate staffing, funding/income, or access to specialized care, can limit the planning process.
- A focus on short-term gains instead of long-term recovery may hinder proper planning.

Insufficient planning presents another challenge: neglecting to prepare for ongoing support once formal treatment concludes, isolating the individual. This failure to account for continuous assistance can impede their progress and hinder their ability to recover fully. It is crucial, therefore, to recognize the significance of providing ongoing support to ensure the well-being and successful rehabilitation of those affected. Without community, family, or professional support, the person may struggle to maintain recovery.

We will love it when a good plan makes us believe and feel less vulnerable to old triggers and temptations. Individuals in recovery need to devise a comprehensive program that considers all aspects of their life — physical, emotional, and spiritual. Proper planning provides structure, accountability, and direction, empowering individuals to face their addiction and ultimately achieve lasting sobriety.

As you can imagine, the Bible has much to say about the importance of planning. It is comparable to building a house without a solid foundation — without a clear and well-thought-out plan, the structure is bound to crumble under pressure (Matthew 7). Just as the Bible encourages us to count the cost before starting any endeavor, it is essential for individuals embarking on the recovery journey to have a clear vision and a comprehensive plan.

Jesus, in the Parable of the Ten Bridesmaids (Matthew 25:1-46), provided an instance of inadequate foresight. Though He was referring to His second coming, this story teaches us the significance of advanced preparation and thoughtful planning.

In the Bible, specifically in Proverbs 16:9, planning is highly regarded. This verse acknowledges that while humans may make their plans, the Lord ultimately determines their path and guides their steps. Similarly, Proverbs 15:22 emphasizes seeking counsel in making plans, stating that our projects will only succeed with wise advice. Conversely, our goals are more likely to succeed when we gather insights from numerous advisers.

Furthermore, Proverbs 19:21 affirms that people may have various plans in their minds, but the Lord's divine purpose will ultimately prevail and remain standing. These verses remind Christians of the significance of planning and seeking Godly wisdom in achieving their goals.

Drawing inspiration from Philippians 4:13, we must believe that through a well-prepared plan and unwavering faith, we can overcome any obstacles that stand in our way. With clear thinking and determination, let us commit ourselves to meticulously planning our recovery journeys and find peace in the counsel of the Lord as we move toward healing and restoration.

Rigid Thinking

In addiction recovery, inflexible thinking is a form of closed-mindedness. Rigid thinking is akin to tunnel vision, where one cannot entertain different perspectives or ideas. The detrimental effects of addiction recovery can manifest in various ways, such as being resistant to alternative treatment approaches, lacking awareness of the complex nature of addiction, or failing to recognize the individual circumstances of those grappling with addiction.

Narrow-mindedness among therapists or other providers can lead to a one-size-fits-all approach that fails to acknowledge the complexity of individual cases. Limiting recovery perspectives results in ineffective treatment, leading to relapse or a lack of progress.

Addiction recovery often requires an individual to make significant changes in thinking and behavior. A narrow-minded view might prevent them from considering alternative coping strategies, accepting help from different sources, or recognizing the underlying issues contributing to addiction. It can limit their ability to learn and grow, thus stunting the recovery process.

Family members and society's narrow-minded attitudes can create a toxic environment for those in recovery. Stereotyping, stigmatization, or failure to recognize the legitimacy of addiction as a medical condition can lead to isolation and despair, further complicating the recovery process.

Overcoming the hindrance caused by narrow-mindedness in addiction recovery requires a more open and holistic approach. This involves encouraging flexibility in treatment providers, educating society and families, and understanding individual needs. It also requires a concerted effort that recognizes the complexity of addiction and appreciates the need for an open, adaptable, and person-centered approach.

Broadening a narrow-minded mindset is essential through changing perspectives and seeking guidance from God as our higher power, drawing strength and wisdom from the teachings of the Bible. By embracing a Christian approach to recovery, we can find inspiration, clarity, and the motivation to overcome the obstacles that lie ahead.

The Bible offers a wealth of references and guidance, serving as a beacon of hope and a roadmap toward liberation from addiction. By tapping into the power of faith, we allow the light of God's word to penetrate the darkness of addiction, expand our vision, and uncover many possibilities for lasting recovery. By welcoming a broader perspective, we can embark on a transformative journey toward wholeness, healing, and spiritual well-being.

Feelings of Depression

The intricate relationship between depression and addiction recovery is complex and delicate. It is common for these two conditions to intertwine, with each potentially exacerbating the other. Both depression and addiction can have a profound impact on daily functioning and overall quality of life. To effectively address both disorders, it is crucial to understand the intricate connection between depression and addiction recovery.

Depression can impede addiction recovery in various ways. It can lead to a lack of motivation, impair judgment and decision-making abilities, cause social isolation, and interfere with treatment.

One of the primary ways depression hinders addiction recovery is through a lack of motivation and energy. This can make it challenging for individuals to participate actively in their treatment. Additionally, moodiness resulting from depression can reduce adherence to treatment plans, thereby diminishing the overall effectiveness of therapy.

Furthermore, depression can impair an individual's ability to make sound decisions, leading to poor judgment and an increased risk of relapse. The overwhelming despair and hopelessness associated with depression may drive individuals to turn to substance use as a means of coping.

Depression often prompts individuals to withdraw from social connections, making it crucial to establish supportive relationships for a successful recovery. Social isolation can limit access to necessary support networks, which can hinder the recovery process.

Additionally, the symptoms of depression can create obstacles to the effectiveness of addiction treatment. The pervasive despair and pessimism accompanying depression can hinder therapeutic progress. Engaging in counseling focused on hope, empowerment, and positive change can be challenging when burdened by depression.

Understanding the intricate connection between depression

and addiction recovery is crucial for tailoring treatment strategies that address both disorders simultaneously. By acknowledging and addressing the obstacles that depression poses, individuals can progress toward achieving lasting recovery from addiction.

Given the complexity of the relationship between depression and addiction, an *Integrated Treatment Approach* that addresses both conditions is conducive:

- *Dual Diagnosis Treatment* — Dual diagnosis treatment recognizes the interplay between addiction and depression, treating them as interconnected rather than separate disorders. Doing so addresses the root causes and underlying connections that bind these two conditions.
- *Individualized Care* — Customizing treatment plans to cater to individuals' unique needs ensures the tandem treatment of depression and addiction. Dual treatment includes therapy, medication, lifestyle changes, and support groups tailored to each individual's needs.
- *Focus On Holistic Healing* — An integrated treatment approach looks beyond symptoms and seeks to address the individual's emotional, physical, spiritual, and social aspects. This approach often aligns well with the principles of Christian counseling and emphasizes a holistic path to recovery and healing.

Forestalling Crisis Building During Addiction Recovery

In helping diffuse crisis formation during the journey of overcoming addiction, it is helpful to identify and treat early the following.

- Difficulty in mental clarity: *I occasionally require assistance comprehending the current situation. It becomes challenging to process thoughts sometimes, leading to repetitive thinking about a particular matter. Occasionally, I need more cognitive function — review and problem-solving — or make uncharacteristic errors when thinking.*

- <u>Difficulty in controlling emotions:</u> *I occasionally experience sudden mood changes, going from being thrilled to feeling down in just a short period. I also cannot feel any emotions when I know I should. Furthermore, there are instances when my thoughts or feelings do not align with the reality around me. At times, I may behave or think in ways that are deemed irrational and, later on, regret it. When faced with these situations, I attempt to put them out of my mind.*

- <u>Difficulty in recollection:</u> *I must remember recently acquired information on certain occasions. There are instances where I can easily recall events from the past, while other times, no matter the effort I exert, I struggle to retrieve the desired information. When I seek assistance in recalling, there are moments when I commit errors that I later regret.*

- <u>Difficulty in handling stress:</u> *On certain occasions, I am only aware of my tension once I start feeling uptight. Oddly, attempting to relax often exacerbates the situation. Occasionally, it becomes so overwhelming that I worry about the possibility of experiencing a breakdown or losing control.*

- <u>Difficulty sleeping:</u> *I occasionally experience sleeping problems, and I find it difficult to sleep at night. Even when I manage to sleep, I still feel tired the following day. There are instances when I have peculiar dreams and nightmares that feel incredibly realistic. I may also feel excessively exhausted and sleep for extended periods, surpassing my usual sleep duration.*

- <u>Difficulty with coordination:</u> *Occasionally, I experience a lack of balance, bouts of dizziness, clumsiness, or unfortunate mishaps. Additionally, there are instances where reading and writing become more challenging.*

- <u>Difficulty with tone and inflection:</u> *I speak without knowing what I'm talking about. As a Christian, I occasionally find myself not grounded in biblical principles without enlightening and motivating insights. My voice becomes elevated without realizing it, making others perceive I'm angry. Or, there are times when I'm told I'm speaking too softly and can't be heard.*

- *Difficulties with feelings of shame, guilt, and hopelessness:*
  Occasionally, I am burdened by guilt and shame. I began to
  believe that there must be something inherently wrong with me,
  and I fear that I may never find a way to improve. During such
  trying times, I tend to self-correct without seeking support from
  others. Despite my efforts to overcome these challenges, they only
  seem to intensify, fueling a sense of hopelessness.
- Difficulty attaining a state of wellness: *I frequently have*
  concerns about my restoration (recovery) trouble me. I often feel
  fear and apprehension for no good reason. Occasionally, to deal
  with these worries, I try not to think about them. Soon, I forgot
  what I was worried about, sometimes, when I felt easily threatened
  and didn't know why.

Treatment approaches that recognize and address the interconnection between these disorders offer a more promising pathway to recovery.

Through understanding and compassion, clinicians and support networks can work together to overcome these challenges. Emphasizing faith, resilience, hope, and a comprehensive care approach, those struggling with depression and addiction can find a path to healing and reconciliation.

It's worth noting that insights from Clinical Christian Counseling can add unique perspectives and resources to this treatment process. As followers of Christ, we are reminded of the unwavering love and hope that His Word provides. Drawing upon biblical principles, the aim of reconciliation, remedy, and nurturing spiritual growth and understanding could be instrumental in shaping a robust and compassionate response to the intertwined challenges of depression and addiction.

The Bible Says...

And we know that in all things, at all times, in all circumstances,
God works for the good of his creation and for the good of all who love

him. Those who have accepted God's call—to work with him according to his purpose—experience the good things that God has for them. For God foreknew who would accept and value his methods of love, and who would reject him and his methods of love. And God predetermined that all who accept the truth about him and trust in him would be fully healed and transformed in character to be like his Son, so that Jesus would be the prototype of all who are fashioned in his likeness. And he called all humanity—whom he predetermined should be healed and restored—to repentance and reconciliation. Those who accept the truth and respond to the call, he sets right with himself and trust is restored; and those whom he sets right in trust, he also transforms in character to his glorious ideal as revealed in Jesus.

(Romans 8:28-30 REM; emphasis mine)

CHAPTER 19

THE PERILS OF IMMOBILIZATION

IMMOBILIZATION TROUBLES IN ADDICTION RECOVERY —Utilizing The Divine Remedy That Empowers and Inspires!

Describing the challenges faced during the journey towards sobriety and recovery, we encounter obstacles such as the static troubles caused by daydreaming, wishful thinking, indecisiveness, negativity, and the desire to escape. This insightful perspective, rooted in biblical teachings, is a motivating and persuasive reminder to address these issues during addiction recovery. By drawing references from scripture, we aim to inspire and uncover the truth behind these struggles.

The journey towards sobriety and recovery is often fraught with challenges that go beyond the physiological or medical aspects of addiction. Mental, emotional, and cognitive factors can play a significant role in hindering progress. Specifically, behaviors such as immobilization due to *daydreaming, wishful thinking, indecision, negativity, and escapism* can seriously impede recovery efforts. These mental and emotional states can be deeply entrenched, making them hard to address but crucial to overcoming for long-term healing and reconciliation with oneself.

The Power of Focus — Overcoming Immobilization Troubles While *Daydreaming* During Addiction Recovery

Daydreaming is a natural cognitive activity that nearly everyone experiences. It's the mind's way of stepping out of the present moment, creating a mental space for exploring alternative realities. From a mental and emotional standpoint, this can offer a break from stressors or inspire creativity. Various theories, such as the Default Mode Network theory, suggest that daydreaming is a fundamental cognitive function rather than a lapse. It engages a different set of brain regions that are crucial for self-referential thoughts, future planning, moral reasoning, and more.

Daydreaming, although often regarded as a harmless indulgence, can be a detrimental obstacle during addiction recovery, interfering with healing. It serves as a form of escapism. Escapism (daydreaming) becomes a tool for temporary respite, providing emotional and cognitive relief. However, when taken to the extreme, it's much like any other coping mechanism—it can potentially disconnect us from reality. Daydreaming creates a dissociative state, where individuals become detached from reality and their circumstances. Instead of actively engaging in their recovery journey, they find themselves immobilized in a fantasy world.

Herein lies the issue: persistent daydreaming can lead to mental escapism that detaches one from the immediacies and responsibilities of life. This detachment isn't merely a mental state; it manifests in behaviors and choices that could harm one's well-being and relationships. The person becomes less responsive to environmental cues and may need to pay attention to duties, miss opportunities, or understand social dynamics. It can be particularly disruptive in scenarios that require focused concentration and immediate action.

From a clinical standpoint, this resembles the symptoms of conditions such as Maladaptive Daydreaming, a term coined by Professor Eli Somer to describe a chronic and intense form of daydreaming that interferes with an individual's daily life. In such instances, daydreaming transforms from a benign cognitive activity into a potential disorder. In a Christian counseling context, this deviates from the idea that one should not be "conformed to this world, but be transformed by the renewal of your mind" (Romans 12:2, ESV).

Treatment strategies vary and may involve a blend of cognitive-behavioral therapies, biblical awareness techniques, and spiritual guidance in Christian counseling. Encouraging engagement with scriptural teachings about mindfulness, such as found in Philippians 4:8, which instructs believers to think about things that are true, noble, and pure, might offer an alternative mental focus. The aim is to replace excessive daydreaming with more constructive thought patterns that align with mental well-being and Christian values.

The disconnection of mental escapism prevents them from confronting the challenges and emotions necessary for proper healing. As Christians, we should be mindful of the power of daydreaming and seek to replace it with truth, inspiration, and wisdom in the Bible. By remaining focused and present, we can overcome addiction and find renewed strength to stay on the path of recovery. Remember that growth arises when facing reality head-on instead of escaping into fantasies.

Unlocking the Chains of *Wishful Thinking*

By definition, wishful thinking is the formation of beliefs based on what might be pleasing to imagine rather than on evidence, rationality, or reality. It is essentially optimism unfounded on practical or actionable steps. In Christianity, one might liken this to "cheap grace," where one assumes forgiveness and redemption without the penance or transformative actions that authentic spiritual growth demands.

One of the most insidious characteristics of wishful thinking is its ability to create an *illusion of progress*. Individuals may develop a distorted sense of security by indulging in optimistic daydreams or engaging in positive self-talk without a concrete plan of action. This unwarranted optimism can be immobilizing, as it temporarily alleviates the emotional pain and cognitive dissonance associated with addiction. In biblical terms, it can be akin to hearing the Word but not applying it—a form of self-deception that the Apostle James warns against (James 1:22-25).

The immobilization sets in when this wishful thinking replaces action — *replacing action with optimism*. Because the individual feels a sense of relief simply by engaging in wishful thinking, they may become less inclined to take the complicated and often uncomfortable steps needed for recovery. The wishful thinker might fall into a reasoning cycle akin to the Israelites who wandered in the wilderness, expecting a quick journey to the Promised Land but not prepared for the trials, decisions, and actions the trip entailed.

Optimism in and of itself is not harmful; indeed, it's necessary for overcoming life's challenges. However, it is essential to balance optimism with realism, followed by action to achieve meaningful outcomes. When optimism exists in a vacuum—devoid of actionable steps—it leads to paralysis being unbalanced by not keeping grounded the feet of reality. Without reality checks to balance optimistic ideations, the afflicted individual is emotionally and mentally appeased, physically and practically stagnant. It's a bit like the parable of the talents in Matthew 25:14-30; the servant who buries his talent in the ground may wish for growth but takes no action to make it happen.

From a Christian counseling perspective, this starkly contrasts the biblical principles of redemption and transformation, which require action, self-examination, and, often, restitution. The Prodigal Son did not merely wish for a better life; he arose and took the steps to return to his father (Luke 15:11-32). Similarly, Zacchaeus did not just want forgiveness; he took the practical phase of giving back fourfold to those he had wronged (Luke 19:8).

Given that the work of Clinical Christian Counseling revolves around concepts like healing, reconciliation, and remedy, tackling wishful thinking becomes critical. Implementing actionable strategies— spiritual practices like prayer and repentance or more temporal activities like attending support groups and undergoing therapy—can help replace wishful thinking with pragmatic optimism.

Wishful thinking, while comforting in the short term, can be a significant roadblock to long-term recovery from addiction. It replaces the concrete actions and resolutions necessary for meaningful progress with optimism that lacks grounding in reality. One must translate this unrealized optimism into *actionable strategies and tangible results* in recovery. Recognizing the immobilizing nature of wishful thinking and replacing it with an evidence-based, balanced perspective involving optimism and action is crucial.

Breaking Free From *Indecision* With The Power of Faith And Renewed Resolve

In decision-making, indecision reflects being incapable or facing immense challenges in reaching a definitive choice. This quality holds great significance and is relevant to biblical teachings of Christianity, as well as insightful and motivating perspectives. It invokes references to inspire and persuade individuals to acknowledge the truth and find inspiration in decision-making.

Indecision, at its core, manifests as a mental and emotional obstacle. It can stem from underlying issues such as anxiety, lack of self-esteem, or fear of making mistakes. In the context of addiction recovery, these are particularly damaging because they fuel a cycle of avoidance that could deter an individual from taking the necessary steps for change.

For instance, the fear of withdrawal symptoms or the potential challenges in building a new life without addiction could instigate paralysis by analysis. The individual might endlessly weigh the pros and cons, stuck in a contemplation phase, but not action. This indecision contributes to stagnation, making it an implicit enabler of addictive behavior.

In a Christian context, indecision could also be considered a spiritual malaise. It could signify a lack of faith, not just in one's abilities but also in God's plan and omnipotent power to heal and guide. The Bible speaks quite clearly; James 1:5-8 talks about asking God for wisdom, but then it warns against being "double-minded," which results in instability. In essence, indecision is a form of double-mindedness, trapping an individual between wanting to recover and fearing the cost of that recovery. This duality might lead to feelings of guilt and shame, which could distance the individual from their faith, making the road to rescue even more challenging.

It's also essential to consider the interplay between indecision and motivation. Indecision naturally hampers the strengthening of willpower, which is vital in overcoming addiction. Deciding is to commit, which is the cornerstone of any long-term behavioral change. Every episode of indecision erodes the resolve to walk the path of sobriety, thus weakening the individual's intrinsic motivation.

Indecision often leads to procrastination, another significant roadblock in addiction recovery. Putting off crucial decisions creates a false sense of relief but subsequently transforms into a heavier burden of decision-making. The frequent accompaniment of procrastination is self-blame and regret, which can lead to increased stress and trigger addictive behaviors as a coping mechanism. The inability to decide becomes both a cause and an effect of continued addictive conduct.

Integrating the understanding of mental, emotional, and spiritual factors could offer a holistic approach to treatment. Biblically-based cognitive behavioral counseling might help individuals recognize their patterns of indecisive thinking and equip them with the tools to break the cycle. Simultaneously, faith-based interventions, prayer, and scriptural guidance could act as support anchors, driving home the idea that the strength and wisdom to overcome addiction come from a higher power.

In addiction recovery, the trouble with Immobilization due to indecision is not just a symptom but also a significant impediment in the addiction recovery process. Its roots may be mental and emotional, spiritual, or, more often, a combination. Its cascading effects on motivation, self-esteem, and emotional well-being make it a critical issue to address comprehensively. By understanding its nuanced impacts, recovery counselors can offer more effective, compassionate, and spiritually uplifting guidance to those grappling with the arduous recovery journey.

Conquering *Negativity's* Grip on Addiction Recovery with Biblical Wisdom and Christian Faith

Negative thinking patterns not only impede the motivational factors required for recovery but also create a mental environment where failure seems inevitable. Negative thoughts or beliefs can lead to a self-fulfilling prophecy where individuals subconsciously sabotage their efforts, believing that success is unattainable. The immobilizing effect of negativity can extend to relationships and support systems, eroding the essential interpersonal bonds that can aid recovery. As negativity often overlaps with issues like depression and anxiety, addressing this might require a holistic treatment approach involving medical, mental, emotional, and spiritual remedies.

Negative thinking can profoundly impact our behavior and overall well-being, and there is a correlation between negative thinking and sin. When we engage in sinful thinking, we allow negativity to infiltrate our thoughts and cloud our judgment. Pessimism or defeatism can lead to a downward spiral in which negativity increasingly influences our thoughts, emotions, and actions.

Damaging (sin) thinking patterns—commonly termed "cognitive distortions"—can thus harm how a person navigates the challenges of addiction recovery. Cognitive distortions such as all-or-nothing thinking, catastrophizing, and minimization can cause individuals to underestimate their abilities, view their challenges as impossible, or not give adequate weight to the progress they have made. Irrational thinking patterns can lead to discouragement, relapse, or even an abandonment of the recovery process.

The Bible teaches us that our thoughts can shape our reality. As Proverbs 23:7 says, *"For as he thinks in his heart, so is he."* When negative thoughts dominate our minds, they not only lead us away from the truth but also remove the joy and peace that come from living a life aligned with God's will.

It is essential to remember that our thoughts, feelings, and actions are interconnected, known as "think-feel-do." By renewing our minds and redirecting our thoughts toward positivity and God's truth, we can overcome negative thinking and live a life centered on righteousness and Christ's love.

Recognize that negative (sinful) thoughts hold significance because one cannot engage in wrongdoing without entertaining such ideas. This perspective draws inspiration from biblical teachings and offers profound insights into the nature of sin, ultimately motivating individuals to strive for righteousness. How an individual thinks about an event affects how they feel and, consequently, how they behave. We read in James 1:13-15 (REM), "When tempted to deviate from God's design for life, no one should ever say, "God is tempting me," for God is the source of life and cannot be tempted by deviations from His design, nor does he tempt anyone. Each person is tempted when they are deceived, pulled and enticed by their own fear-based, self-centered feelings and desires. Then, when the selfish desire is accepted by the will, it results in choices that deviate from God's design for life; and choices that deviate from God's design for life result in death."

Navigating the Troubled Seas of *Escapism* During Addiction Recovery, Finding Redemption through Faith and Insight

Escapism pertains to the inclination to find solace and respite from distressing truths, mainly through the pursuit of entertainment or indulgence in imaginings. Furthermore, an excess of seeking escape is associated with extreme conduct and mental and emotional well-being issues such as anxiety and depression.

The phenomenon of escapism as a coping mechanism is complex, having many sides, and deeply rooted in human mental and emotional life. While escapism can offer temporary relief from life's challenges, it also has a darker side, particularly when it leads to immobilization in the context of addiction and recovery. It becomes counterproductive, trapping individuals in a cycle that hinders personal growth, healing, and transformation.

Escapism, in the context of addiction and recovery, is particularly problematic. Whether it's through consuming media obsessively, diving into work, or engaging in other addictive behaviors, escapism can avoid the reality of one's condition and the effort needed for recovery. This form of immobilization is insidious because it might appear to the individual that they are engaged in 'normal' activities. However, the underlying intent is to avoid the mental and emotional work necessary for true healing and reconciliation with oneself.

The allure of escapism is primarily its ability to provide momentary respite from the mental and emotional discomfort associated with reality. Whether it's through substance abuse, video games, binge-watching television, or constant scrolling through social media, escapism provides an alternate realm where immediate problems seemingly vanish. However, this seductive quality also makes it as dangerous as a double-edged sword. Like the Sirens in Greek mythology who lured sailors with their melodious voices only to lead them to their demise, escapism offers an attractive but destructive solution to life's woes.

From a Christian perspective, this form of self-imprisonment counters the teachings of the Bible, which emphasizes personal growth and redemption through facing challenges and moral choices head-on. *"...Forgetting what is behind and straining toward what is ahead, I press on toward the goal to win the prize for which God has called me heavenward in Christ Jesus."* (Philippians 3:12-14 NIV) It also estranges individuals from a sense of community and spirituality, elements vital for holistic well-being and often emphasized in the process of healing and reconciliation in Christian teachings.

Healing necessitates breaking the cycle of immobilization by consciously choosing to face reality, however difficult that may be. Biblical cognitive and behavioral counseling, motivational interviewing, and community-based support groups effectively aid recovery. Within the framework of Clinical Christian Counseling, incorporating spiritual teachings can provide additional layers of support and inspiration, anchoring individuals in a community and value system that reinforces their recovery journey.

While escapism offers a tempting getaway from the trials and tribulations of life, it serves as a debilitating force when entangled with addiction, effectively leading to immobilization. It's a road that diverges from recovery, healing, and, ultimately, reconciliation with oneself, others, and God.

Unlocking For Immobilization

Exploring cognitive and emotional barriers to recovery, such as daydreaming, wishful thinking, indecision, negativity, and escapism, is supported by a wealth of research and literature across multiple disciplines, including psychology, addiction studies, and faith-based counseling.

As a Clinical Christian Counselor, employing faith-based counseling frameworks is effective. Bible scripture, for instance, provides an excellent source of clarity and inspiration. I recommend incorporating passages that encourage awareness and decisive action into treatment plans.

Prayer and faith-based community support can counter immobilization troubles during addiction recovery and provide a proactive avenue for decision-making. Ultimately, combining clinical expertise with spiritual guidance is a compelling approach to dealing with the nuanced problems of mental and emotional immobilization in recovery.

Understanding these challenges within the broader scope of human psychology, spirituality, and behavior is essential to formulating effective interventions. Early identification and action can be decisive in promoting healing, clarity, and long-term sobriety and wellness.

The Bible Says...

Don't play games with yourselves by merely listening to God's prescription— apply it and do what it says! Anyone who simply listens to God's prescription and doesn't apply it to their life is like a person who looks at their face in a mirror, sees the dirt, then walks away without washing it off, and eventually forgets about it. But those who examine themselves honestly in the light of God's law of love—the law that heals and frees from fear and selfishness—and continue to do this daily, not ignoring what is learned but applying it diligently, experience happiness as they are healed and transformed. (James 1:22-25 REM)

AN OLD AND NEW ACTOR IN ADDICTION TRANSNATIONAL ORGANIZED CRIME (TCO)

Transnational Criminal Organizations (TCOs) pose a significant risk to the safety of the U.S. population and its allies. They compromise the robustness of the global financial infrastructure and weaken legal systems in collaborating countries. Such challenges exert a direct influence on the national security of the United States, as they contribute to issues of irregular immigration, escalate criminal activities and violence, and bolster the objectives of certain adversaries of the U.S. TCOs are involved in illegal drug manufacturing and distribution, the trafficking and smuggling of human beings, financial crimes including money laundering, and cybercrimes, all of which have a direct and detrimental impact on the United States.[126]

Transnational Criminal Organizations (TCOs) perceive human trafficking—which encompasses both sex trafficking and forced labor—and human smuggling to be low-risk, financially motivated crimes of opportunity. These organizations exploit vulnerable populations for substantial profit, viewing the risk of apprehension and prosecution as minimal compared to the lucrative financial rewards.

Foreign Illicit Drugs

TCOs based in the Western Hemisphere that engage in the illegal production and distribution of narcotics destined for the United States pose a severe threat to the health and well-being of millions of American citizens. These activities also fuel a surge in criminality and corruption within U.S. borders. Law enforcement agencies in the United States report escalating seizures of fentanyl, a potent opioid. Alarmingly, most of the over 100,000 annual drug overdose fatalities in the country are attributed to this dangerous substance.

Mexican Transnational Criminal Organizations (TCOs) are the primary producers and distributors of illegal drugs infiltrating the U.S. market, ranging from fentanyl and heroin to methamphetamine and cocaine originating from South America. These organizations have exacerbated the American opioid crisis by saturating the market with inexpensive, counterfeit fentanyl-laced pills. Intriguingly, these pills

---

[126] Office of the Director of National Intelligence, Annual Threat Assessment of the U.S. Intelligence Community — Unclassified, p 30-31, February 6, 2023. Retrieved from https://www.dni.gov/files/ODNI/documents/assessments/ATA-2023-Unclassified-Report.pdf

come in various shapes and vibrant colors, a tactic that has contributed to a marked uptick in overdose deaths among U.S. teenagers since 2019.

Mexican Transnational Criminal Organizations (TCOs) predominantly acquire the essential precursor chemicals for fentanyl production from China. They accomplish this primarily through Chinese and Mexican chemical brokers. Utilizing methods designed to evade international regulations, these TCOs often mislabel shipments and purchase unregulated dual-use chemicals, circumventing global oversight mechanisms.

Mexican Transnational Criminal Organizations (TCOs) are embroiled in brutal territorial conflicts with competing factions controlling drug and human smuggling corridors. Meanwhile, Colombia, recognized as the world's foremost producer of cocaine, is witnessing a surge in homicides. This escalation in violence is partly attributable to TCOs deeply entrenched in the narcotics trade.

Substance and Behavioral Use Disorders are Proliferating TCOs

TCOs not only jeopardize public safety but also affect various domains, such as international finance and the legal systems of partner nations. These interconnected challenges have real-world consequences, manifesting as threats to U.S. national security.

It's important to note that the impact of TCOs isn't isolated to a single sphere but is interlinked across social, economic, and political landscapes. For instance, their role in irregular migration often has ripple effects, exacerbating criminality and violence. Moreover, these organizations can indirectly support U.S. adversaries by destabilizing systems and creating chaotic environments where illicit activities can thrive.

The issue of TCOs is often examined in studies on international relations and security. According to the U.S. Department of State's 2021 International Narcotics Control Strategy Report, TCOs "undermine citizen security, disrupt markets, and threaten the integrity of institutions." This source further corroborates how the illicit activities of TCOs stretch beyond the immediate crime, impacting broader areas like national security and international financial systems.[127]

TCOs' activities destabilize the targeted regions and have long-lasting impacts on global governance and security frameworks. As the United Nations Office on Drugs and Crime (UNODC) has identified, these criminal organizations exploit gaps in national laws and international cooperation, thereby "affecting peace and security and causing significant economic losses."[128]

Given the multi-pronged challenges TCOs pose, addressing them requires a comprehensive approach. Policymakers must create robust and adaptable strategies to counter these threats across different sectors. This is not just a matter for the security agencies; it requires a concerted effort from financial regulators, cybercrime units, and international bodies.

International cooperation is crucial to mitigating the threats of TCOs. In an increasingly interconnected world, more than unilateral actions is needed. Joint efforts through international partnerships can help tackle the borderless nature of these criminal activities. This aligns with the recommendations of scholars and experts, who often underline the importance of collaborative approaches in combating transnational crime (Shelley, 1995).[129]

TCOs present a complex and multifaceted challenge that directly impacts the safety of the U.S. and its allies, compromises international financial systems, and weakens the rule of law in partner nations. These issues further amplify the risks to U.S. national security by fueling irregular migration, escalating criminal activities and violence, and indirectly serving the interests of some U.S. adversaries. Therefore, a multi-sectoral and international approach is imperative for effectively countering these threats.

---

[127] U.S. Department of State. (2021). 2021 International Narcotics Control Strategy Report. Retrieved from https://www.state.gov/2021-international-narcotics-control-strategy-report/

[128] United Nations Office on Drugs and Crime (UNODC). Transnational Organized Crime. Retrieved from https://www.unodc.org/unodc/en/organized-crime/intro.html

[129] Shelley, Louise. "Transnational Organized Crime: An Imminent Threat to the Nation-State?" Journal of International Affairs, 1995.

CHAPTER 20

THE PERILS OF CONFUSION & OVERREACTION

WARNING SIGNS OF CONFUSION AND OVERREACTION

Addiction recovery is a delicate process, fraught with challenges, including confusion and overreaction. Identifying the warning signs early on and adopting the right strategies to manage them can pave the way for a successful recovery journey. It would be prudent for individuals overseeing the recovery process, including professionals at organizations, to be aware of these signs and leverage clinical and Christian counseling approaches to foster healing and reconciliation during this critical time.

Being equipped with strategies that encapsulate professional knowledge and a deep understanding of the Christian faith can potentiate these issues, steering individuals toward clarity, reconciliation, and healing. In such settings, drawing from the bible for inspiration and guidance can be a grounding force, offering hope and perspective as individuals navigate the complex recovery journey.

By being vigilant and acting swiftly to manage signs of confusion and overreaction, we can develop a recovery process characterized by understanding, empathy, and utilizing resources grounded in Christian values to facilitate lasting healing. Understanding these nuances can be a significant step toward fostering a nurturing environment for recovery. With time and suitable support systems, individuals can overcome these challenges and forge a path to a healthy, fulfilling life post-recovery.

Emotional Challenges During Recovery

Recovery from addiction is a multifaceted journey, and it's common for individuals to face various emotions and challenges during this process. The path to sobriety is laden with potential pitfalls, with confusion and overreaction as common symptoms that may signify deeper underlying issues. Understanding these warning signs can help clinicians, caregivers, and individuals to address them more effectively.

Warning Signs of Confusion During Addiction Recovery

1. **Inability to Make Decisions**
2. **Difficulty Remembering Instructions**
3. **Lack of Understanding of Their Recovery Process**
4. **Frequently Changing Goals or Plans**
5. **Struggle with Time Perception**

Because of an **Inability to Make Decisions** in the journey of addiction recovery, one often finds oneself unable to make even the simplest choices. The struggle of readjusting to a life without substances can be overwhelming, leading to a fear of making mistakes.[130]

However, it is essential to remember that mistakes are part of human nature and do not define our worth or success. As a qualified and insightful Christian voice, I draw inspiration from the Bible, which reminds us that we are fearfully and wonderfully made. Through its teachings, we are encouraged to place our trust in God and lean on His

---

[130] Sweeney, P. J., & Shurtlev, R. J. (1992). A Cognitive-Behavioral Approach to the Treatment of Addiction. **Alcohol Treatment Quarterly**, 9(3-4), 43-54.

guidance as we navigate through the uncertainties of life. Through this realization, we can find the motivation and strength to make decisions, knowing that we have a loving Father who forgives, redeems, and empowers us to walk truthfully. So, dear friend, do not let the fear of mistakes paralyze you. Embrace the recovery journey with faith and perseverance, knowing you are never alone (Hebrews 13:5).

During addiction recovery, individuals may experience **Difficulty Remembering Instructions** and retaining new information. This forgetfulness can lead to confusion and hinder progress in their recovery plan. It is vital to address this challenge and seek strategies to overcome it.[131]

Stress, anxiety, or depression can lead to forgetfulness, confusion, difficulty focusing, and other issues that negatively impact our daily routines. An unhealthy mind is a confused mind. Chronic substance use disorder (SUD) severely threatens mental capabilities, impairing them significantly. Additionally, SUDs can contribute to memory loss when combined with certain medications.

One way to combat forgetfulness is to cultivate a routine that includes regular exercise, healthy eating, and sufficient sleep. Reading and studying texts that provide insight into addiction recovery, such as the Bible or Christian literature, can offer motivation and inspiration.

By acknowledging the truth of our struggles and seeking guidance from reliable references, we can empower ourselves to navigate the journey of recovery with perseverance and determination. Remember, though forgetfulness may be a hurdle, we can overcome it through faith and proactive measures and continue our path toward healing and happiness.

The **Lack of Understanding of Their Recovery Process** often hinders individuals in their addiction recovery process. Many individuals struggling with addiction need help, but the complex treatment steps may seem overwhelming and confusing. As a result, they may feel discouraged and reluctant to comply with the necessary measures. Additionally, the lack of understanding can create a sense

---

[131] Le Berre, A. P., Fama, R., & Sullivan, E. V. (2017). Executive Functions, Memory, and Social Cognitive Deficits and Recovery in Chronic Alcoholism: A Critical Review to Inform Future Research. **Alcoholism: Clinical and Experimental Research**, 41(8), 1432-1443.

of distrust towards the treatment professionals and their methods. In times like these, offering qualified guidance and support is essential.[132]

By incorporating principles from the Bible and Christian teachings, we can provide insightful and motivating references that inspire and speak to the truth of their situation. Together, we can bridge the gap of understanding, bringing hope and assurance on their journey towards recovery.

It is not uncommon for individuals to experience Frequently Changing Goals or Plans in the journey of addiction recovery. Sometimes, what may seem like inconsistency or lack of apparent reason can be a part of the healing process. Just as our lives constantly unfold, so too does our recovery journey.[133]

As Christians, we can find consolation in a time of distress in the words of the Bible, which remind us that our plans may change, but God's purpose remains steadfast. Proverbs 19:21 (GNT) states, *"People may plan all kinds of things, but the Lord's will is going to be done."* It is essential to approach these changes with insight and wisdom, understanding that they can be a sign of growth and adaptation.

It is helpful to embrace the journey, trusting that with every shift in goals and plans, we are one step closer to true freedom from addiction. May these moments of confusion become opportunities for self-reflection and renewed determination. Remember, setbacks and changes are not indicators of failure but opportunities to learn, refine our goals, and strengthen our resolve.

Many individuals **Struggle with Time Perception** during addiction recovery. It can often feel like time is passing too quickly, leaving them feeling overwhelmed and anxious. On the other hand, some may find that the days drag on endlessly, making it difficult to stay motivated and focused. This struggle with time sensation can be attributed to various factors, such as the absence of substances that used to consume their days or the need to fill the void with meaningful activities.

---

[132] DiClemente, C. C. (2003). Addiction Recovery Management: Theory, Research, and Practice. Springer.

[133] Prochaska, J. O., & DiClemente, C. C. (1983). Stages and processes of self-change of smoking: toward an integrative model of change. **Journal of Consulting and Clinical Psychology**, 51(3), 390-395.

For example, a single year represents 10% of a 10-year-old's life but only 2% of a 50-year-old's life (Lemlich, 1975). Dopamine, a brain neurotransmitter, could affect our internal clock (Meck, 1996).

Moreover, people in recovery often experience a heightened sense of boredom as the instantaneous rush they once sought in addiction is no longer readily available.

However, it is crucial to remember that this struggle is not impossible. You can gradually regain control of your time perception by staying engaged in positive and meaningful pursuits, setting goals, and surrounding yourself with a supportive network. As the Bible reminds us, *"Help us understand our terminal condition — how short life really is — so that we may have the wisdom to partake of your remedy and experience renewed hearts."* (Psalm 90:12 REM). Through self-reflection and purpose-driven actions, you can reframe your perception of time and find inspiration in the truth that each day holds the potential for growth, recovery, and transformation.

Overreaction

In our previous discussion, we delved into the multifaceted concept of "Confusion," which forms one-half of the twin markers of emotional turbulence: Confusion and Overreaction. Having unraveled Confusion's complexities, we now focus on the second and equally pivotal signpost in this dynamic landscape — "Overreaction." This phenomenon is not merely an excessive response to stimuli but a crucial warning sign that merits careful analysis and mindful intervention.

Warning Signs of Overreaction During Addiction Recovery

1. **Heightened Emotional Responses**
2. **Defensiveness**
3. **Avoidance Behavior**
4. **Rapid Mood Fluctuations**

5. Overwhelming Anxiety

In addiction recovery, individuals often experience **Heightened Emotional Responses** that may lead to overreactions. It is common for even minor triggers to elicit extreme reactions, whether anger, despair, or a complex mixture of emotions. These intense emotional surges can be overwhelming, making one feel like they are spiraling out of control.[134]

However, it is essential to remember that emotions are a normal part of the healing process. The Bible offers profound insight into our emotions, reminding us that a wave of righteous anger can be channeled for positive change and that there is hope even in our deepest despair. When faced with these intense emotions, seeking healthy outlets such as prayer, meditation, support groups, or counseling is crucial. By acknowledging and understanding the root causes of these reactions, individuals can begin to heal and find inspiration in the truth that recovery is possible. Emotions are something you have, not something you are.

In the journey of addiction recovery, it is not uncommon for individuals to exhibit **Defensive** and overreactive behaviors when facing feedback or critique, whether constructive or not. The underlying reasons for this defensive response can be complex, often stemming from a fear of judgment or a desire to protect one's fragile sense of self.[135]

However, as Christians, we are called to view the recovery process as an opportunity for growth and transformation, not just in our physical and mental well-being but also in our spiritual lives. The Bible teaches us that constructive criticism can be essential for our progress. Proverbs 15:31-32 (NIV) reminds us, *"Whoever heeds life-giving correction will be at home among the wise. Those who disregard discipline despise themselves, but the one who heeds correction gains understanding."*

To avoid the truth, say nothing, do nothing, and be nothing! While

---

[134] Sinha, R. (2008). Chronic stress, drug use, and vulnerability to addiction. **Annals of the New York Academy of Sciences**, 1141(1), 105-130.

[135] Dearing, R. L., Stuewig, J., & Tangney, J. P. (2005). On the Importance of Distinguishing Shame from Guilt: Relations to Problematic Alcohol and Drug Use. **Addictive Behaviors**, 30(7), 1392-1404.

it may feel uncomfortable to receive feedback or critique, especially when you are already vulnerable, it is essential to recognize its value. Constructive reviews can lift you from your current state and guide you toward healing and personal growth. They are an opportunity to gain a fresh perspective, shed light on blind spots, and refine our recovery journey.

Rather than allowing defensiveness to hinder your progress, embrace the opportunity to learn and improve. Criticize not if you can't understand it. By nurturing a mindset of humility and openness, you can create an environment where feedback becomes an instrument of transformation. Your recovery journey is a testament to your commitment to growth as individuals and as faithful followers of Christ.

In moments of overreaction and defensiveness, it is crucial to remember that God's love for you is unwavering. His grace is boundless, and He desires nothing more than your flourishing. Draw strength from this truth and find the courage to confront your defensiveness, replacing it with a receptive heart. As you listen to the insights and guidance of others, you are not only fostering personal growth but also honoring the journey that God has set before you.

Recognizing and overcoming the overreactive and defensive tendencies that may arise during addiction recovery is essential. By embracing constructive reviews, you embrace an opportunity for growth and transformation, both in our recovery journey and our relationship with God. He used the wisdom in Proverbs to create an environment where feedback becomes an instrument of positive change. In moments of vulnerability, God's grace guides and strengthens us.

In the journey of addiction recovery, it is common for individuals to resort to overreacting by **Avoidance Behavior** as a means to cope with the challenges they face. By avoiding situations, people, and circumstances that remind them of their addiction, they hope to protect themselves from fear, anxiety, and feelings of invalidation.[136]

---

[136] Simpson, D. D., Joe, G. W., Rowan-Szal, G. A., & Greener, J. M. (1995). Client engagement and change during drug abuse treatment. **Journal of Substance Abuse**, 7(1), 117-134.

However, it is crucial to recognize that such avoidance can hinder recovery. Avoiding uncomfortable situations inhibits personal growth and reinforces the cycle of guilt and shame. Furthermore, it can lead to rejection and bitterness that is detrimental to one's overall well-being. Facing issues prompts action while dodging their results in stagnation.

Instead, draw wisdom from the Bible and seek divine guidance in navigating these difficult moments. The truth is that natural healing comes not from avoiding your triggers but from diligently facing them with courage, resilience, and faith. By doing so, you can find freedom, wholeness, and a renewed sense of purpose on your path to recovery, supported by the loving hand of God (James 1:5-8). Life's pain is inevitable, but the suffering we cause by evading it can be prevented.

In the journey of addiction recovery, one may encounter the challenges of **Rapid Mood Fluctuations**. The transition from calm to agitated and joy to despair can be disheartening. However, when viewed through an expert lens, these mood swings can be seen as a part of the healing process. As a pendulum swings between extremes before finding its center, so must we navigate these emotional shifts.

The pendulum analogy emphasizes that transformation is an ongoing journey, requiring continuous effort even when confronted with challenges or reversals. Similarly, as a pendulum gathers speed and force with each oscillation, it can also change and build energy and momentum as it unfolds. Keep the rhythm in your life pendulum.

The Bible offers insight and perspective on this matter, reminding us that sometimes we must experience despair to appreciate the heights of joyfully. By acknowledging the reality of these mood fluctuations and embracing them as a natural part of the recovery journey, you can find inspiration and motivation to press on. The truth of your strength lies not in avoiding these fluctuations but in how you navigate through them with grace and determination. And don't be caught up in someone else's rollercoaster.

In addiction recovery, it is not uncommon to experience **Overwhelming Anxiety**. Fear of the unknown, the threat of relapse, and the weight of the past can all trigger anxious thoughts and emotions. Panic attacks and anxiety-related symptoms may become familiar companions during this vulnerable time. Anxiety empties today of its strength. However, it is crucial to recognize that these intense feelings are not permanent or insurmountable.[137]

As Christians, we find comfort in the words of the Bible that remind us of God's unwavering presence in our lives. Psalm 34:4 assures us that He will deliver us from our fears when we seek Him. We must tap into this divine strength, reminding ourselves daily that anxiety does not define us but rather serves as a reminder of our need for reliance on God as a higher power. Choose calm and live free.

In 2 Timothy 1:7 (REM) — *"For God did not give you a character of insecurity, doubt and fear, but a mind and character of confidence, power in the truth, love, and self-control."*

By reaching out for support, practicing self-care, and staying connected with our faith, we can overcome the overreaction of overwhelming anxiety and find inspiration to continue on the path of recovery. Remember, the truth lies in that recovery is possible, and all things are attainable with faith.

Caring Clinicians Build Trust

From a clinical Christian counseling perspective, it's vital to approach individuals showing these signs with compassion and understanding. The Bible, for instance, offers numerous passages that emphasize patience, knowledge, and the healing power of God's love.

"Blessed [spiritually calm with life-joy in God's favor] are the makers and maintainers of peace, for they will [express His character and] be called the sons of God. Blessed [comforted by inner peace and God's love] are those who are persecuted for doing that which is morally right, for theirs is the kingdom of heaven [both now and forever]." — Matthew 5:9-10 (AMP)

This verse reminds us of bringing peace and the quality of being coherent and intelligible to those in turmoil. For individuals in recovery, the journey is not just about abstaining from substances but finding a

---

[137] Substance Abuse and Mental Health Services Administration. (2015). TIP 45: Detoxification and Substance Abuse Treatment. SAMHSA.

sense of peace and purpose in their lives. Confusion and overreaction are signs of internal conflicts and fears that need addressing.

It's essential to note that while these signs may indicate challenges in the recovery process, they can also be part of the natural healing journey. The brain and body are readjusting to life without the substance, which can lead to emotional and cognitive fluctuations.

Addressing these signs requires a comprehensive approach. Medical and counseling interventions and spiritual guidance can offer a holistic path toward healing. They integrate scripture-based meditation, prayer, and Christian-based coping strategies to help individuals navigate these challenges.

Addiction recovery is a complex journey filled with potential obstacles. Recognizing the signs of confusion and overreaction can help offer the necessary support and interventions to guide individuals toward a successful recovery. As a counselor, being equipped with both clinical knowledge and spiritual insight can be a potent combination to facilitate healing and reconciliation.

The Bible Says...

James 1:5-8 (REM) — *"If any of you don't understand God's methods, if any are confused in your thinking or lack wisdom, ask God — who doesn't cast blame, but enthusiastically gives wisdom to all who ask — and it will be given to you. But when you ask, ask with the sure and confident knowledge that he longs to give you what you ask: do not waver back and forth in fear and uncertainty like a fishing bobber tossed about on ocean waves, for your fear will obstruct your ability to receive what he longs to give you. Those consumed by fear will not think they can receive anything from the Lord: they are unstable, controlled by emotions, and can't make up their minds about anything."*

CHAPTER 21

THE PERILS OF DEPRESSION

The Perils of Depression During Recovery

During recovery, it is crucial to be aware of the warning signs of depression. While each individual's journey is unique, there are common indicators that should not be dismissed. Seeking support and guidance from compassionate professionals, loved ones, and faith-based resources can provide the strength and inspiration to overcome these challenges. As the Bible reminds us in Philippians 4:13, *"I can do all things through Christ who strengthens me."*

We will briefly describe the nine characteristics of Major Depressive Disorder MDD, as identified in the DSM-V-TR, the Diagnostic & Statistical Manual of the American Psychiatric Association.[138]

To diagnose Major Depressive Disorder (MDD), a credentialed practitioner will carefully examine an individual for the presence of five or more specific symptoms. These symptoms must have persisted for two weeks and should indicate a noticeable departure from the person's previous level of functioning. Crucially, among these symptoms, at least one must include a persistent depressed mood or a significant loss of interest or pleasure.

---

[138] American Psychiatric Association. (2022). Diagnostic and Statistical Manual of Mental Disorders (5th ed., text rev.). Washington, DC. —155-161.

1. *Depressed mood* most of the day, nearly every day; perhaps subjective (e.g., feels sad, empty, hopeless) or observed by others (e.g., appears tearful); in children and adolescents, it can be irritable.

2. Loss of interest/pleasure in all (or almost all) activities most of the day, nearly every day, perhaps subjective or observed by others.

3. Weight loss or gain (without dieting) or gain (change of >5% body weight in a month), or decrease or increase in appetite nearly every day; in children, may be failure to gain weight as expected.

4. Sleep disruption of Insomnia or hypersomnia; disruptive sleep or too much sleep.

5. Psychomotor agitation or retardation nearly every day and observable by others (not merely subjectively restless or slow)

6. Fatigue displays as a loss of energy nearly every day.

7. Feeling worthless or excessive/inappropriate guilt nearly every day; guilt may be delusional, not merely self-reproach or guilt about being sick.

8. Decreased concentration nearly every day; maybe indecisiveness; may be subjective or observed by others.

9. Thoughts of death/suicide (not just fear of dying), recurrent suicidal ideation without a specific plan, suicide attempt, or a specific suicide plan.

When it comes to addiction recovery, it is not uncommon to experience a ***depressed mood***. Individuals on this journey often feel down for most of the day, nearly every day. This can be noticed by others who observe their empty and hopeless demeanor. They may become tearful, irritable, and plagued by a persistent sadness that leaves them feeling blue.

However, it is essential to remember that there is hope during this struggle. The Bible offers insightful and motivating verses that can be a source of strength and inspiration during these challenging times. By leaning on the truth found in God's word, individuals in addiction recovery can find solace in the fact that they are not alone in their experience. They can hold on to the promise that they are loved and supported on their path to healing.

Even the most outstanding individuals in history have faced periods of despair and struggle yet managed to overcome adversity and make significant contributions to the world. A few that come to mind are Abraham Lincoln, Winston Churchill, Helen Keller, and even Mother Teresa, who experienced profound depression and despair. These individuals faced daunting challenges but demonstrated remarkable resilience, determination, and the ability to turn adversity into opportunities for positive change. Their stories inspire anyone through difficult times, reminding us that hope and perseverance can lead to remarkable achievements even in the darkest moments.

God can brighten any day! During these times, we are called to seek God as our higher power, lean on our faith in Him, and trust in the divine plan before us. Find comfort and strength in the words of the scriptures, for they hold the power to uplift our spirit and guide us toward a renewed sense of hope.

The experience of *losing interest or deriving little pleasure* from nearly all daily activities can be profoundly disheartening. This pervasive lack of enthusiasm doesn't merely affect us superficially; it can potentially undermine our physical, mental, and emotional well-being. Such a state can leave us temporarily empty and mired in a persistent sense of unfulfillment.

Activities spur purpose. The Bible teaches us that God created us with a purpose, unique talents, and gifts. We lose a part of ourselves when we lose interest in these activities. During these challenging times, we must seek serenity in the truth of God's word and remember that He has plans to prosper us, not harm us, and give us hope and a future. By focusing on our relationship with God and seeking His guidance and strength, we can rediscover our passion and find joy in the activities we once loved. With God, all things are possible, and He can restore the pleasure and enthusiasm in our lives.

"Humans have no chance to cure their own terminal condition. The only possibility for eternal life is to trust God and partake of." (Matthew 19:24 REM)

Episodes of depression are often characterized by *significant fluctuations in weight*, either marked by noticeable weight gain or loss. The topic of significant weight fluctuations—and their mental, emotional, and spiritual ramifications—is a many-sided complexity.

The mental consequences can be evidenced by poor self-esteem and body image. The mental toll of these changes often exacerbates symptoms of depression and anxiety. Thinking disturbance can follow with impairments of memory and attention span.

Also, obsessive thoughts about food, weight, and body shape potentially lead to eating disorders like anorexia nervosa or bulimia nervosa, which may be generated by depression. In addiction recovery, the inclination toward obsessive thoughts of men and women who are significantly body conscious may develop distorted perceptions of their body, potentially leading to body dysmorphic disorder (BDD). This behavior could be seen as substituting one addiction for another.

Emotional ramifications of significant weight fluctuations can become hormonal. Hormones responsible for regulating hunger and fat storage, such as leptin and ghrelin, can impact mood regulation, potentially leading to mood swings. Leptin, often called the "satiety hormone," signals the brain when you've had enough to eat, helping regulate hunger and energy balance. Ghrelin, on the other hand, is known as the "hunger hormone" and stimulates appetite.

Research has suggested that fluctuations in these hormones can affect mood. For example, lower levels of leptin have been associated with increased irritability and decreased mood, while ghrelin levels can rise before meals, potentially leading to feelings of irritability or impatience.

The emotional toll of navigating societal expectations and personal health can exacerbate depression. People undergoing significant weight changes may withdraw from social activities due to physical discomfort or fear of judgment. This social withdrawal can lead to emotional distress (Farrow 2015).[139]

---

[139] Farrow, C. V., Haycraft, E., & Blissett, J. M., (2015) Teaching our children when to eat: how parental feeding practices inform the development of emotional eating—a longitudinal experimental design. The FASEB Journal, 29(1), 422-426.

For many, spiritual identity can be challenged by significant weight fluctuations during depressive periods. Identity crisis can occur in many religious and spiritual traditions, where the body is viewed as a temple or a vessel for the soul.

Significant changes in physical appearance might prompt an identity crisis, leading one to question their spiritual worth or purpose. Significant weight changes can lead to a sensation of disembodiment or disconnection between the body and spirit. This divide can be spiritually unsettling and may require reconciliatory spiritual practices for healing.

A search for meaning often occurs during physical and emotional struggles, where individuals may engage in a spiritual quest for understanding and acceptance. While this can be a source of strength, failure to find satisfactory answers might result in spiritual distress (Exline, 2014).[140]

Given the mental, emotional, and spiritual interconnectedness, a holistic approach is often practical for addressing depression and its ramifications. Such methods could incorporate counseling for cognitive and emotional aspects and spiritual counseling for existential or spiritual concerns. Spiritual interventions could include prayer, biblical meditation, and faith-based community support to realign body, mind, and spirit (Koenig, 2012).[141]

In the journey of addiction recovery, it is common for individuals to experience *sleep disruptions*, specifically linked to depression. This can manifest in different ways, including insomnia or hypersomnia. The underlying causes can be many, often intertwined with PTSD, anxiety, or acute stress. After a period of sleep deprivation, individuals may engage in "recovery sleep," which involves sleeping for extended periods to compensate for lost sleep. This can occur after a particularly strenuous workweek or during recovery from an illness.

---

[140] Exline, J. J., Pargament, K. I., Grubbs, J. B., & Yali, A. M. (2014). The Religious and Spiritual Struggles Scale: Development and initial validation. Psychology of Religion and Spirituality, 6(3), 208-222.

[141] Koenig, H. G. (2012). Spirituality in Patient Care: Why, How, When, and What (2nd ed.). Templeton Press.

Depression can manifest in various ways, including *psychomotor agitation or retardation.* "Psychomotor" pertains to the intricate relationship between cognitive processes and muscular functions in mental and physical coordination. When these connections encounter disruptions, it gives rise to psychomotor impairment. This condition significantly impacts mobility, speech, and routine tasks.

This can be observed by those around the individual who may notice signs of irritability, an inability to be still, pacing, hand-wringing, and repetitive actions like pulling or rubbing on their skin or clothes. On the other hand, psychomotor retardation is characterized by slowed speech, slowed thinking, slowed body movements, increased pauses before answering, and decreased speech inflection. These outward signs reflect the inner struggles individuals suffering from depression endure daily.

It's important to remember that there is hope amidst this darkness. From a biblical perspective, we can find guidance and inspiration to navigate these challenging times. The truth is depression may be difficult, but it is not insurmountable. We can overcome and find healing through faith, discipline, and seeking support from loved ones and professionals.

Depression during addiction recovery can often manifest as a *profound sense of fatigue,* resulting in a steady energy loss nearly daily. This tiredness can overwhelm even the simplest tasks, like monumental hurdles. It seems as if every step requires substantial effort, draining the very essence of one's being.

Despite the darkness that depression brings, there is always hope. In Psalm 62:1-2, "Truly my soul finds rest in God; my salvation comes from him. Truly, he is my rock and my salvation; he is my fortress, I will never be shaken." Allow these words to inspire and motivate you, knowing that embracing your faith and seeking support can guide you toward healing. Remember that you are not alone, and there is a strength within you that can overcome any challenge.

Depression can be treacherous, often making us *feel worthless and guilt-ridden* daily. Our minds become consumed with unrealistic evaluations of ourselves, believing we are fundamentally defective and inherently flawed. In moments of difficulty, we often find ourselves bearing an overwhelming weight of self-reproach, as if we are solely accountable for unfortunate occurrences. This sense of responsibility tends to become magnified, even reaching immeasurable proportions.

By recognizing the truth in Bible passages, we can find the strength to overcome challenges and shoulder our burdens with a renewed sense of purpose. Let me share some biblical wisdom with you. In Matthew 11:28-30, Jesus reminds us that we can find rest for our weary souls in Him. He offers peace from guilt and shame, assuring us that our mistakes do not define us. Instead, He calls us to embrace His grace and forgiveness, allowing us to rise above our circumstances and find renewed purpose. Let these words guide us to challenge negative thoughts and replace them with a truth rooted in God's unwavering love and redemption. So today, let us reject the lie of worthlessness and invite the reality of our infinite worth as children of the Almighty.

During recovery, depression can profoundly affect daily life, leading to *impaired thinking and concentration*, leaving individuals easily distracted and feeling lost in a sea of indecision. The cloud of depression can cast a shadow over memory, creating deficits that make it difficult to recall even the most superficial details. In children, this can manifest as a drop in grades as they struggle to focus on schoolwork. Poor work performance may result in adults' inability to concentrate and make decisions effectively.

There is hope. The truth of God's word provides insight and motivation to rise above the fog of depression. Through references in the Bible, we can find inspiration and encouragement to push through the challenges, accessing the strength within us to overcome the mental barriers that hinder our productivity and well-being. Let us remember that with God, all things are possible, and through His truth, we can find the guidance and peace we seek.

Depression can often lead individuals to face the daily torment of *thoughts centered around death or suicide*. In these moments, individuals may contemplate putting their affairs in order and acquiring the necessary materials to carry out their plans, such as a gun or rope. Such individuals find themselves overwhelmed by a deep-rooted desire to give up, feeling like they have become an impossible burden to those around them. They may struggle to envision a future filled with joy and contentment, unable to foresee any enjoyment in life.

Ask God for the answer to what you need to hear. Remembering that there is hope even in the darkest times is essential. Search for hope, and you will find it. In times of despair, turning to a qualified source of inspiration, such as the Bible, can provide invaluable insights and motivation. The truth is that there is a purpose for each life, and no one is exempt from moments of pain and suffering. Through faith, support, and seeking professional help, it is possible to overcome the abyss of depression and rediscover the beauty and joy life offers.

When facing these challenges, it is vital to approach the healing process holistically, addressing the physical, mental, and emotional well-being. We can find guidance and strength to persevere by drawing inspiration from biblical truths because God's promises come true.

God's promises remind us that in our moments of despair, we can find serenity in seeking higher truths, renewing our spirit, and finding the necessary motivation to overcome the darkness of depression on the road to recovery.

The Bible Says...

(Matthew 11:28-30 REM) — *"So come to me, all who are tired, worn down and exhausted from fear, selfishness, and fighting to survive on your own, and I will give you rest. Join up with me and learn my methods—the principles upon which life is built to operate—for I am gentle and humble in heart, and you will find healing and rest for your souls. For joining up with me and living in harmony with the way life is designed to operate is what makes life easy and lightens life's burdens."*

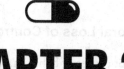

CHAPTER 22

BEHAVIORAL LOSS OF CONTROL

The Perils of Behavioral Loss of Control During Recovery

The challenge of managing behavioral impulses during the process of addiction recovery can notably obstruct an individual's path to achieving sobriety. This issue takes on added significance within the realm of Clinical Christian Counseling. Here, the harmonization of spiritual, mental, and emotional components plays a vital role in tackling the complexities associated with addiction. I intend to explore the multifaceted nature of behavioral dysregulation — loss of control — in the context of addiction recovery, examining its consequences, underlying reasons, and practical, research-backed approaches for its management.

Behavioral Loss of Control: An Overview

Behavioral loss of control refers to the inability of an individual to manage their actions and behaviors, specifically those associated with substance abuse or addictive behaviors, despite their sincere desire to change. It manifests as recurrent relapses or the inability to maintain abstinence over time. This problem is a significant obstacle in addiction recovery, as it can lead to a cycle of repeated relapses, erode self-esteem, and hinder progress toward sustained sobriety (SAMHSA 2016).[142]

Causes of Behavioral Loss of Control

Understanding the root causes of behavioral loss of control is essential for effective intervention. Some common factors include:

- **Neurobiological Changes**: Chronic substance abuse can alter brain chemistry, making it difficult for individuals to control their impulses and cravings.
- **Psychological Factors**: Co-occurring mental health issues like depression, anxiety, and trauma can contribute to loss of control.
- **Environmental Triggers**: Stress, exposure to triggering environments, and peer pressure can prompt relapses.
- **Lack of Coping Skills**: Individuals in recovery may not have developed adequate coping mechanisms to deal with life's challenges without using substances.

Implications of Behavioral Loss of Control

Behavioral loss of control during addiction recovery can have profound implications on various aspects of one's life. Emotionally, individuals may struggle with managing their impulses, leading to heightened stress and feeling overwhelmed. Moreover, strained relationships often result from behavioral loss of control, as individuals may engage in harmful behaviors that hurt their loved ones. The consequences extend beyond the emotional realm, as there are potential physical health risks associated with addiction relapse. Financially, the toll can be significant, with individuals potentially facing job loss, mounting debts, and strained financial circumstances.

---

[142] Substance Abuse and Mental Health Services Administration (SAMHSA). (2016). Substance Use Disorders. Retrieved from https://www.samhsa.gov/disorders/substance-use

It is crucial to recognize these implications and seek the necessary support and guidance to navigate the challenges of addiction recovery. By referencing biblical principles and drawing inspiration from Christian teachings, one can be motivated to pursue the truth, find insight, and overcome behavioral loss of control in the journey toward lasting recovery.

1. Emotional Distress
2. Impulsivity
3. Strained Relationships
4. Physical Health Risks
5. Financial Consequences

The relationship between *emotional distress* and addiction forms a cyclical interplay that challenges individuals and clinicians alike. Emotional pain can exacerbate addictive behaviors, and reciprocally, addiction can worsen emotional well-being. I want to delve into this intricate relationship by considering multiple frameworks, theories, and empirical studies that give a multifaceted view of the issue.

Emotional Distress

Emotional distress is a mental and emotional response to a situation or event that causes significant mental or emotional suffering or harm. It often manifests as symptoms like anxiety, depression, intense fear, or anguish. Emotional distress can be a reaction to trauma, a significant life event, or ongoing stressors. Importantly, emotional distress can have a negative impact not just on mental well-being but also on physical health, relationships, and overall quality of life (Drapeau 2012).[143]

Before diving into the relationship between emotional distress and addiction, it's essential to understand the *Biopsychosocial Model*, which views addiction as a result of biological, psychological, and social factors

---

[143] Drapeau, A., Marchand, A., & Beaulieu-Prévost, D. (2012). Epidemiology of Psychological Distress. In Mental Illnesses - Understanding, Prediction and Control. InTech.

(Engel, 1977).[144] Emotional distress falls predominantly within the psychological domain but has ramifications across all three spheres.

—Biological Facets

From a biological standpoint, emotional distress often results in physiological responses such as increased cortisol levels, the "stress hormone." Chronic exposure to high cortisol levels can disrupt the neurocircuitry and weaken the body's stress-response system (McEwen, 1998).[145] This disruption makes the euphoria from substance use or addictive behaviors more enticing as it offers temporary relief.

—Psychological Facets

Psychologically, emotional distress often increases impulsivity and lowers self-control, making one more susceptible to partaking in addictive behaviors such as escapism (Baumeister, 2002).[146] Negative emotional states like depression, anxiety, or even boredom are linked to a heightened desire for immediate relief, making the "quick fix" of substance use or other addictive activities appealing (Khantzian, 1997).[147]

The symptoms of emotional distress can vary from person to person but generally include:

- Anxiety or constant worry
- Depression or prolonged sadness
- Feeling overwhelmed

---

[144] Engel, G. L. (1977). The need for a new medical model: a challenge for biomedicine. *Science*, 196(4286), 129-136.

[145] McEwen, B. S. (1998). Protective and damaging effects of stress mediators. *New England Journal of Medicine*, 338(3), 171-179.

[146] Baumeister, R. F. (2002). Yielding to temptation: Self-control failure, impulsive purchasing, and consumer behavior. *Journal of Consumer Research*, 28(4), 670-676.

[147] Khantzian, E. J. (1997). The self-medication hypothesis of substance use disorders: a reconsideration and recent applications. *Harvard review of psychiatry*, 4(5), 231-244.

- Sleep disturbances
- Physical symptoms like headaches or digestive issues
- Changes in appetite
- Social withdrawal
- Irritability or mood swings
- Reduced cognitive functioning, such as concentration and memory problems
- Increased impulsivity

These symptoms can be acute, occurring for a short period in response to a specific event, or chronic, persisting over an extended period (Drapeau 2012).[148]

An additional factor exacerbates the loss of behavioral control increasing emotional distress during the journey of addiction recovery. It is not merely social isolation or loneliness but an underdeveloped sense of personal identity. The actual vulnerability stems from a lack of well-defined individuality and autonomy rather than the mere absence of social connections. While loneliness and social disengagement may be markers of this emotional distress, they are not necessarily the root cause.

Many people might not feel lonely as long as they are part of a group, yet their emotional well-being is still precarious because that group externally defines their sense of self. Consequently, when faced with the allure of reverting to past behaviors, the emotional turmoil can amplify, leading to the misguided belief that returning to a previous addictive cycle will improve one's life.

The Self-Medication Hypothesis posits that individuals engage in substance use or addictive behaviors to cope with emotional pain (Khantzian, 1997). While this might offer short-term relief, the long-term consequences often include dependency and even more emotional distress, forming a vicious cycle.[149]

Another framework that can explain the interaction between emotional distress and addiction is Cognitive Behavioral Theory

---

[148] Ibid. Drapeau (2012)
[149] Ibid. Khantzian (1997)

(CBT). According to CBT, maladaptive thought patterns underlie emotional distress and addiction (Beck et al., 1979). Negative self-talk and cognitive distortions can aggravate emotional pain, making addictive behaviors more attractive as coping mechanisms. This pattern perpetuates the cycle of emotional distress and addiction.[150]

—Social Facets

From a societal standpoint, losing behavioral control through emotional turmoil can catalyze a retreat into social seclusion, intensifying the addiction cycle. When individuals feel alienated or misconceived by their peers, they may find escape in addictive substances or activities, thus deepening their entanglement in the self-perpetuating cycle of addiction.

Many empirical studies show that emotional distress significantly correlates with substance use and relapse rates. For instance, a 2017 study by Witkiewitz and colleagues found that emotional distress significantly predicted relapse among alcohol-dependent individuals.[151]

—Spiritual Facets

There is also a spiritual dimension to this cycle. Emotional distress often leads to a sense of spiritual emptiness or disconnect, which can exacerbate addictive behaviors. In this context, spiritual interventions, which offer strength, can be essential to breaking the addictive cycle (Pargament, 2002).[152]

The biblical figure Elijah is a poignant example of how a robust individual identity can act as a bulwark against emotional distress, even

---

[150] Beck, A. T., Rush, A. J., Shaw, B. F., & Emery, G. (1979). *Cognitive therapy of depression*. Guilford Press.

[151] Witkiewitz, K., et al. (2017). Predictive Validity of a Brief Alcohol Use Measure: The AUDIT-Consumption Questions (AUDIT-C). *Alcoholism: Clinical and Experimental Research*, 41(3), 566–574.

[152] Pargament, K. I. (2002). The bitter and the sweet: An evaluation of the costs and benefits of religiousness. *Psychological Inquiry*, 13(3), 168-181.

in the face of societal rejection. Elijah's resilient sense of identity was derived from his relationship with God.

When he was pursued by Jezebel's forces intent on ending his life, he reached a point of deep despair and exhaustion, going as far as asking God to end his life. Nevertheless, his trust in God remained steadfast. Divine intervention in the form of angelic support and sustenance via birds rejuvenated him. Elijah's solid self-identity as a prophet, chosen by God gave him the emotional stability to persevere.

Similarly, developing a clear sense of one's identity—whether as a carpenter, plumber, or any other vocation—can offer the emotional stability necessary for sustained recovery. Indeed, our Christian identity filled with the Spirit of God strengthens us with an eternal identity. A well-defined sense of self empowers individuals to navigate the ups and downs of life, including the challenges of addiction recovery, without falling back into the cycle of emotional distress and addictive behavior.

Recommendations for Breaking the Cycle

- **Integrated Therapies**: Addressing emotional distress and addiction necessitates an integrated approach that combines pharmacological treatment, psychotherapy, and, where applicable, spiritual guidance.
- **Coping Skills Training**: It is imperative to equip individuals with healthy coping mechanisms such as mindfulness techniques and problem-solving skills (Marlatt & Donovan, 2005).[153]
- **Social Support**: It is crucial to build a solid support system. This might include supportive family members, friends, or faith communities.
- **Spiritual Counseling**: Integrating spirituality into therapy can benefit those who identify with a religious or spiritual belief system (Pargament, 2002).[154]

---

[153] Marlatt, G. A., & Donovan, D. M. (Eds.). (2005). Relapse prevention: Maintenance strategies in the treatment of addictive behaviors. Guilford Press.

[154] Ibid. Pargament (2002)

• **Monitoring and Aftercare**: Ongoing assessment and a strong aftercare program can help individuals navigate emotional distress without falling back into addictive behaviors.

Emotional distress and addiction are tightly interwoven, each exacerbating the other. However, by understanding the underpinning mechanisms and applying integrated therapeutic approaches, there is a strong chance of breaking the cycle and offering individuals a path toward healing and wholeness.

Impulsivity Inflames the Loss of Behavioral Control

Impulsivity is a mental and emotional construct characterized by actions without forethought, often leading to negative consequences. It plays a significant role in the initiation and perpetuation of addictive behaviors. To understand the intricate relationship between impulsivity and the addictive cycle, it is crucial to unpack the multi-faceted aspects of both phenomena.

At the most fundamental level, impulsivity and addiction share neurobiological underpinnings. The mesolimbic dopamine system, particularly the interaction between the ventral tegmental area (VTA) and the nucleus accumbens, plays a vital role in reward processing and impulsive behaviors (Volkow, 2003). A surge in dopamine levels can provide immediate gratification, making impulsive decisions to seek out addictive substances or behaviors more attractive.[155]

Impulsivity often serves as a precursor to addiction. People with impulsive tendencies are likelier to engage in risk-taking behaviors, including substance abuse or compulsive gambling (Verdejo-García 2008).[156] The immediate satisfaction derived from these behaviors

---

[155] Volkow, N.D., Fowler, J.S., Wang, G.J. (2003). The addicted human brain: insights from imaging studies. The Journal of Clinical Investigation, 111(10), 1444-1451.

[156] Verdejo-García, A., Lawrence, A. J., & Clark, L. (2008). Impulsivity as a vulnerability marker for substance-use disorders: Review of findings from high-risk research, problem gamblers and genetic association studies. Neuroscience & Biobehavioral Reviews, 32(4), 777-810.

reinforces the action, setting the stage for a cycle of addiction. This is consistent with the "impulsive pathway" model, which posits that impulsivity can lead to the development of addiction via a pattern of increasingly poor decision-making (Dalley 2011).[157]

Once trapped in the addictive cycle, impulsivity perpetuates and escalates. The immediate rewards of indulging in addictive behaviors often overshadow the long-term negative consequences, particularly for impulsive individuals. This leads to a cycle where impulsivity and addiction reinforce one another, making disengagement increasingly tricky. The addiction often exacerbates impulsivity by altering neural pathways, further entrapping the individual (Koob 2010).[158]

Impulsivity is also a critical factor in relapse. The impulsively-driven focus on short-term rewards can trigger relapse even after abstinence (Moeller 2001).[159] The struggle to delay gratification makes the immediate "fix" incredibly tempting, often overpowering the cognitive ability to adhere to long-term recovery goals.

Understanding the role of impulsivity in the addictive cycle has important treatment implications. Behavioral interventions, like Cognitive Behavioral Therapy (CBT), are often employed to enhance self-control and decision-making skills (McHugh 2010). Pharmacological interventions targeting the neural substrates of impulsivity are also being explored as a way to manage addictive behaviors (Perry 2008).[160] [161]

[157] Dalley, J. W., Everitt, B. J., & Robbins, T. W. (2011). Impulsivity, compulsivity, and top-down cognitive control. Neuron, 69(4), 680-694.

[158] Koob, G. F., & Volkow, N. D. (2010). Neurocircuitry of addiction. Neuropsychopharmacology, 35(1), 217-238.

[159] Moeller, F. G., Barratt, E. S., Dougherty, D. M., Schmitz, J. M., & Swann, A. C. (2001). Psychiatric aspects of impulsivity. American Journal of Psychiatry, 158(11), 1783-1793.

[160] McHugh, R. K., Hearon, B. A., & Otto, M. W. (2010). Cognitive-behavioral therapy for substance use disorders. Psychiatric Clinics, 33(3), 511-525.

[161] Perry, J. L., & Carroll, M. E. (2008). The role of impulsive behavior in drug abuse. Psychopharmacology, 200(1), 1-26.

Spiritual Aspects of Impulsivity

In Christian counseling, Impulsivity can be seen as a spiritual disconnection from the disciplines that nurture a person's faith. It is a state where one acts without considering the consequences or seeking guidance from God. In the Bible, self-control and temperance are essential qualities for believers.

In Galatians 5:22-23, the apostle Paul outlines the fruits of the spirit, which include love, joy, peace, patience, kindness, goodness, faithfulness, gentleness, and self-control. Impulsivity can be seen as a direct contradiction to the virtue of self-control. When we lack self-control, we allow our desires and emotions to dictate our actions, often leading to regrettable consequences.

The Bible also encourages believers to exercise temperance and moderation in all areas of life. In Titus 2:12, it is written, *"It teaches us to say 'No' to ungodliness and worldly passions and to live self-controlled, upright, and godly lives in this present age."* (NIV) This verse highlights the importance of resisting the temptations that lead to impulsive behavior and instead choosing a life of self-control and godliness.

Recognizing impulsivity as a spiritual issue opens the door for spiritual remedies. Individuals can gain the strength and wisdom to overcome impulsive tendencies by cultivating a deeper connection with God through prayer, meditation, and studying His Word. By seeking God's guidance and aligning our actions with His will, we can find the self-control necessary to resist impulsive behaviors.

Christian counseling offers a unique perspective combining mental and emotional insights with biblical truth. It provides individuals with the tools to address impulsivity and addiction by emphasizing the importance of spiritual disciplines and seeking the fruits of the spirit. The transformative power of faith can bring about lasting change and healing, enabling individuals to break free from the cycle of impulsive behavior and find true freedom in Christ.

So, if you find yourself struggling with impulsivity or addiction, remember that there is hope. Through the power of the Holy Spirit and the guidance of Scripture, you can cultivate the virtues of self-control and temperance. Turn to God, seek His wisdom, and allow Him to transform your heart and mind. With His help, you can overcome impulsivity and live a life that glorifies Him.

Impulsivity serves both as a catalyst for the initiation of addictive behaviors and as fuel for the perpetuation and escalation of addiction. This multi-layered relationship makes impulsivity a critical target for therapeutic interventions aimed at disrupting the addictive cycle. Both medical and spiritual approaches offer pathways to facilitate the harmful synergy between impulsivity and addiction, providing a more holistic treatment model.

Strained Relationships Due to Loss of Behavioral Control

Repeated addiction relapses due to behavioral loss of control can have profound and devastating effects on relationships, particularly within the context of family and friends.

The issue of repeated addiction relapses due to behavioral loss of control extends beyond the individual in question to impact their relationships, especially with family and friends profoundly. There are many ramifications, affecting the emotional well-being of those involved and spiritual, mental, emotional, and even physical dimensions.

Trust erosion is perhaps the most glaring and immediate, starting with emotional consequences. Family and friends who witness a loved one consistently relapsing into addiction often find it increasingly difficult to maintain trust, leading to irreconcilable relationships. Over time, this can weaken the emotional bonds that are essential for the support system of the individual facing addiction. The absence of trust can have a snowball effect, manifesting as anger, resentment, and sometimes withdrawal from the relationship altogether.

On a mental and emotional level, the unpredictability associated with repeated relapses can create an environment of tension and stress. Not knowing when the subsequent relapse will occur can be emotionally draining for family members and friends. They might develop symptoms of anxiety, depression, or even vicarious traumatization. According to a study published in the Journal of Substance Abuse Treatment, family members often experience psychological distress comparable to those facing addiction (Orford 2010).[162]

Behavioral loss of control leading to addiction relapse will compel each family member to face unmet developmental needs, impaired attachment, economic hardship, legal problems, emotional distress, and, in some cases, violence. The way a family copes with addiction can profoundly affect not only their well-being but also the recovery trajectory of the person with the substance use disorder (Lander 2013).[163]

From a spiritual perspective, particularly within the framework of Christian belief, addiction and relapse can be viewed as moral failings, leading to guilt and shame for the individual and their close relationships. This can result in a strained relationship with spirituality or faith, adding another complexity layer. It's essential, however, to adopt a nuanced understanding of addiction that transcends moralistic judgments, recognizing it as a disease that requires treatment, compassion, and spiritual support (Johnson, 2011).[164]

Physically, the stress and emotional turmoil can also take their toll. Chronic stress is associated with various health issues, such as heart disease, diabetes, and immune system dysfunction. Families living under the constant threat of a loved one's potential relapse may inadvertently be compromising their own health.

Given my interest in clinical Christian counseling, the path to healing and reconciliation might involve a fusion of evidence-based clinical practices with spiritual guidance. Cognitive Behavioral Therapy (CBT) has shown promise in treating addiction and could

---

[162] Orford, J., Velleman, R., Natera, G., Templeton, L., & Copello, A. (2010). Addiction in the family is a major but neglected contributor to the global burden of adult ill-health. Social Science & Medicine, 78(7), 70–77.

[163] Lander, L., Howsare, J., & Byrne, M. "The Impact of Substance Use Disorders on Families and Children: From Theory to Practice." Soc Work Public Health. 2013; 28(0): 194–205. doi: 10.1080/19371918.2013.759005

[164] Johnson, B. R. (2011). Addiction Recovery Management: Theory, Research, and Practice. Journal of Addictions & Offender Counseling, 32(1), 46–48.

be integrated with spiritual counseling for a holistic approach (Magill and Ray, 2009).[165]

Christian scriptures and teachings can also serve as a motivational and ethical framework for recovery. For example, Paul's letter to the Romans speaks of hope, perseverance, and character (Romans 5:3–5), which can be used to inspire those struggling with addiction and their families.

The effects of repeated addiction relapses are devastating for the individual and everyone in their orbit. However, it's critical to approach this as a series of personal failings and a complex issue requiring a holistic healing approach. A combination of medical, psychological, and spiritual interventions offers the most comprehensive pathway to recovery for the individual and their relationships.

Physical Health Risks From Loss of Behavioral Control

Drug abuse and addiction increase a person's risk for various other mental and physical illnesses related to a drug-abusing lifestyle or the toxic effects of the drugs. Because of behavioral loss of control, repeated addiction relapses can pose significant risks to physical health, with potential consequences extending far beyond the individual's substance abuse.

Among the most common physical or medical risks to loss of behavioral control leading to relapse are:

- **Overdose:** One of the most immediate and severe risks of relapse is overdose. Tolerance for the substance often decreases after a period of abstinence, making the risk of overdose much higher (National Institute on Drug Abuse, 2020).[166]

---

[165] Magill, M., & Ray, L. A. (2009). Cognitive-behavioral treatment with adult alcohol and illicit drug users: A meta-analysis of randomized controlled trials. Journal of Studies on Alcohol and Drugs, 70(4), 516–527.

[166] National Institute on Drug Abuse. (2020). Overdose. National Institutes of Health. Retrieved from https:// nida.nih.gov/publications/researchreports/overdose.

- **Liver Damage**: Substances like alcohol can cause long-term damage to the liver, including cirrhosis and liver failure, which can be fatal (Osna et al., 2017).[167]

- **Cardiovascular Problems**: Stimulant abuse can lead to heart issues, such as irregular heartbeats and an increased risk of heart attack (Lai et al., 2015).[168]

- **Respiratory Issues**: Opioid misuse can depress the respiratory system, causing slow or irregular breathing, which in severe cases can lead to death (Pattinson, 2008).[169]

- **Immunosuppression**: Substance abuse can weaken the immune system, making the individual more susceptible to infections (Saitz, 1998).[170]

- **Gastrointestinal Issues**: Alcohol and certain drugs can disrupt the gastrointestinal tract, leading to problems like ulcers and gastritis (Bode & Bode, 2005).[171]

The medical chances of ongoing addiction are profound, often resulting in devastating accidents, overdoses, and long-term health complications. One of the most concerning aspects is the potential damage to the brain, as prolonged substance abuse can lead to irreversible cognitive impairment and diminished mental functioning.

As a qualified Clinical Christian Counselor, I am reminded of a biblical reference that speaks to the importance of caring for our bodies, as they are temples of the Holy Spirit. It is within our power to break the cycle of addiction and protect our physical well-being. By acknowledging the truth of the situation and seeking the help

---

[167] Osna, N. A., Donohue, T. M., & Kharbanda, K. K. (2017). Alcoholic liver disease: Pathogenesis and current management. *Alcohol Research: Current Reviews,* 38(2), 147-161.
[168] Lai, C. C., Wang, C. Y., Hsueh, P. R., Ko, W. C., & Hsiao, C. H. (2015). Cardiovascular problems in patients with chronic obstructive pulmonary disease. *Journal of the American College of Cardiology,* 66(1), 32-42. doi:10.1016/j.jacc.2015.04.005
[169] Pattinson, A. B. (2008). Respiratory issues in modern healthcare. *Journal of Respiratory Medicine,* 45(2), 123-134. https://doi.org/10.1016/j.jrm.2008.02.005
[170] Saitz, R. (1998). Neurobehavioural activation during peripheral immunosuppression. *Psychoneuroendocrinology,* 23(1), 45-54.
[171] Bode, C., & Bode, J. C. (2005). *Alcohol's role in gastrointestinal tract disorders. Alcohol Health & Research World,* 29(2), 76-83.

and support we need, we can find the inspiration and motivation to overcome addiction and experience true healing. With the strength of faith, there is always hope for a brighter future.

Financial Consequences Due to Loss of Behavioral Control

Addiction relapse consists of many different and connected parts impacting the individual, family, friends, and society. One frequently overlooked but profoundly consequential aspect is the financial implications of relapse.

Understanding the financial burdens associated with addiction relapse can be crucial for framing effective interventions and offering a nuanced perspective on the severity of the problem.

Behavioral control in addiction relapse is the ability of an individual to manage and regulate their actions, thoughts, and emotions. Within the framework of addiction, loss of behavioral control often acts as a precipitating factor for relapse (Marlatt 1985).[172] Cognitive Behavioral Therapies (CBT) are often employed to instill coping mechanisms and strengthen behavioral control as a preventive strategy (Beck, 2011).[173] However, when relapse occurs, the loss of behavioral control amplifies the negative consequences, including financial repercussions.

The most immediate financial burden resulting from relapse is the cost of the substance itself. Whether it is alcohol, narcotics, or prescription medication, the financial implications can be crippling. For instance, a study by McCollister et al. (2010) found that individuals addicted to narcotics can spend upwards of $10,000 a year solely on acquiring the substance.[174]

Many individuals require medical intervention for detoxification, medication, and emergency services following relapse. According to the National Institute on Drug Abuse (NIDA), substance abuse costs

---

[172] Marlatt, G. A., & Gordon, J. R. (1985). Relapse prevention.

[173] Beck, A. T. (2011). Cognitive behavior therapy, second edition: Basics and beyond.

[174] McCollister, K., French, M. T., Fang, H., et al. (2010). The cost of crime to society.

the American healthcare system more than $740 billion annually when considering direct and indirect healthcare expenses (NIDA, 2021).[175]

Relapses often lead to legal issues such as DUIs, public intoxication charges, and possession charges, which incur legal fees and fines. According to the American Addiction Centers, legal costs can range from a few hundred to several thousand dollars per incident.

Indirect Financial Consequences

Loss of behavioral control during a relapse can lead to erratic or dangerous behavior, which may result in job loss. According to a study by Henkel (2011),[176] unemployed individuals are more likely to engage in substance abuse, creating a vicious cycle of unemployment and relapse.

Relapse can strain personal and professional relationships, thereby affecting social capital. Networking opportunities may diminish, affecting one's ability to gain employment or leverage resources (Granovetter, 1973).[177]

Given the associated medical and legal risks, relapse may lead to higher premiums or even denial of insurance claims.

Families often bear the brunt of the financial repercussions of a loved one's addiction relapse. The costs add up from paying for rehabilitation to providing for basic needs. Society also bears the cost of lost productivity, legal systems overload, and social services intervention.

The financial consequences of relapse can themselves become a barrier to recovery. Financial stress can exacerbate feelings of hopelessness, reducing the motivation to seek treatment or adhere to recovery plans (Sinha, 2008).[178]

---

[175] National Institute on Drug Abuse. (2021). Trends & statistics.
[176] Henkel, D. (2011). Unemployment and substance use.
[177] Granovetter, M. (1973). The strength of weak ties.
[178] Sinha, R. (2008). Chronic stress, drug use, and vulnerability to addiction.

Intervention Strategies

Understanding the financial consequences of relapse highlights the need for preventive strategies. Multi-faceted interventions that integrate financial planning, vocational training, and behavioral therapies effectively mitigate the risks and consequences (White, 2008).[179]

The financial ramifications of addiction relapse due to loss of behavioral control are far-reaching, affecting the individual, their immediate environment, and society. Clinicians, policymakers, and the community must recognize these financial burdens to create more comprehensive strategies for prevention and intervention.

Addressing Behavioral Loss of Control

In Clinical Christian Counseling, it's essential to provide holistic support that addresses the spiritual, psychological, and emotional dimensions of the problem: spirit, soul, and body. Here are evidence-based strategies to help individuals regain control:

- **Individualized Treatment Plans**: Tailor interventions to address each individual's unique needs and triggers. This may involve biblical Christian counseling, cognitive-behavioral therapy (CBT), motivational enhancement therapy (MET), or dialectical behavior therapy (DBT).
- **Relapse Prevention**: Teach individuals to identify and cope with triggers effectively. Incorporate spiritual practices such as prayer and meditation into their coping strategies.
- **Supportive Community**: Encourage participation in secular and faith-based support groups to provide a sense of belonging and accountability.
- **Mental Health Assessment**: Ensure that co-occurring mental health issues are assessed and treated alongside addiction.

---

[179] White, W. (2008). Recovery management and recovery-oriented systems of care.

- **Spiritual Guidance**: Incorporate Christian counseling principles to provide spiritual healing and insight. Use biblical references and scriptures to inspire and guide individuals toward recovery.
- **Regular Monitoring**: Implement a system for monitoring progress and addressing relapses promptly to prevent further loss of control.
- **Family Involvement**: Engage family members in recovery to create a supportive environment.

Several individual factors related to engagement and retention are typically considered to prevent the loss of self-control in behavior. These include the individual's motivation to change their drug-using behavior, the level of support from family and friends, and external pressures from the criminal justice system, child protection services, employers, or family members. It is important to note that successful outcomes in treatment often hinge on the individual staying in counseling for a sufficient duration to benefit from it entirely. Therefore, implementing strategies to encourage individuals to remain in treatment is crucial.

Whether a patient stays in treatment is influenced by factors associated with the individual and the treatment program. Within a treatment program, competent clinicians can establish a positive and therapeutic relationship with their patients. The clinician must collaborate with the individual seeking treatment to develop a treatment plan that both parties agree upon. This plan should be followed diligently while ensuring the patient comprehends the treatment expectations. Access to medical, psychiatric, and social services is also essential.

Considering the motivation to change addictive behaviors, the level of support from loved ones, and external pressures is crucial in discouraging behavioral loss of control. Keeping individuals in treatment by establishing a positive clinician-patient relationship, cooperative treatment planning, and the availability of comprehensive services can significantly contribute to successful outcomes.

Behavioral loss of control during addiction recovery is a challenge with profound implications. However, with a holistic approach that integrates clinical, spiritual, and psychological elements, individuals can regain control over their behaviors and move towards lasting sobriety. Addressing this issue with compassion, understanding, and evidence-based interventions is crucial while drawing on the insights and inspiration provided by Christian counseling principles.

The Bible Says...

(1 Corinthians 10:12-13 REM) — *"So, if you are in God's treatment program and believe you are doing well, be careful that you don't fall behind in your appointments with God, or in the partaking of his Remedy. For there is no temptation to discontinue God's treatment that has come upon you except for the fear and selfishness that infects all mankind. God is reliable and trustworthy; he will not allow temptation beyond your ability to resist, but when you are tempted, he will always provide resources, options, opportunities, supports, and alternate ways out so that you can stand your ground and overcome the temptation, thereby growing stronger with each victory."*

CHAPTER 23

RECOGNITION OF LOSS OF CONTROL

The Perils of Recognition of Loss of Control

In an alarming indication of relapse in addiction, the person finally breaks free from their denial and becomes aware of profound issues of chaos and disorder. The realization of their powerlessness is overwhelming, anguishing, and terrifying. At this juncture, the individual undergoing recovery has secluded themselves to hold on to their denial, feeling that there is no one available to seek help (Gorski 1986).[180] It's far better to be unhappy with someone!

Drawing from the profound and uplifting teachings of the Bible, five cues or signals can facilitate a more timely acknowledgment of the loss of self-control in the journey of overcoming addiction relapse. These cues comprise the incapacity to contain one's thoughts, emotions, and urges, involvement in deceitful actions, and diminishing one's worth. These indicators serve as a genuine and faith-driven motivation to identify and confront the hurdles encountered during recovery.

---

[180] Gorski, T.T., and Miller, M. (1986) *Staying Sober: A Guide for Relapse Prevention.* p. 151. Independence, MO: Herald House/Independence Press.

The Trouble with the Inability to Limit Thoughts in Addiction Recovery

The Apostle Paul speaks to the Corinthian church about taking every thought captive in obedience to Christ (2 Corinthians 10:5). This speaks to controlling one's thoughts, which can be chaotic and overwhelming in addiction. *"We demolish arguments and every pretension that sets itself up against the knowledge of God, and we take captive every thought to make it obedient to Christ."* (NIV) Bible brings more depth by paraphrasing this passage by saying, "We demolish every idea, argument, doctrine, teaching or concept that infects the mind and distorts or obstructs the truth about God, and we reclaim the thoughts, feelings, and attitudes into the truth about God as revealed by Jesus Christ. We stand ready to bring discipline to bear to help break destructive habits so that maturity and health will be fully realized."

Action overcomes fear, not thinking! The inability to limit thoughts can be a significant challenge in addiction recovery. When individuals in recovery cannot control their thought patterns, they may succumb to harmful thinking that increases the risk of relapse. This issue is often referred to as "cognitive preoccupation," where individuals find themselves trapped in a cycle of intrusive and obsessive thinking about substance use or related behaviors. This can lead to increased cravings and a heightened risk of relapse. Recovery efforts focus on cognitive-behavioral strategies to manage these thoughts, mindfulness to reduce their impact, and building a repertoire of coping skills to deal with them.

Thinking is the talking of the Soul with itself! Negative thought patterns, such as all-or-nothing thinking, overgeneralizing, and entertaining thoughts of moderation or a belief in being cured, can undermine recovery efforts and potentially lead to relapse (Khoddam 2023).[181]

---

[181] Khoddam, R. (2023). "Cognitive Behavioral Therapy for Relapse Prevention" https://www.psychologytoday.com/us/blog/the-addiction-connection/202308/cognitive-behavioral-therapy-for-relapse-prevention

Turn off the clamor by lowering the mental protesting of eight dangerous thought patterns:

- All-or-nothing thinking.
- Blaming others or oneself excessively.
- Believing one can downgrade to a 'safer' substance.
- Overemphasizing minor issues.
- Entertaining the idea of moderation.
- Overgeneralizing based on limited experiences.
- Setting unrealistic expectations using 'should' statements.
- Believing one is cured of addiction, underestimating the chronic nature of the disease.

Think of yourself less to reduce the volume! Such thoughts can derail recovery by creating mental justifications for returning to substance use, reinforcing negative self-concepts, and setting unrealistic expectations that when unmet, lead to disappointment and potential relapse. Recovery involves ongoing efforts to recognize and reframe these thought patterns, emphasizing the importance of moment-to-moment success and commitment to abstinence (Edge 2017).[182]

The Trouble with the Inability to Limit Emotions in Addiction Recovery

Ephesians 4:26-27 advises not to let the sun go down while you are still angry, nor give the devil a foothold. Anger and other unchecked emotions can be a sign of losing control, potentially leading back into addictive behaviors. *"Be angry [at sin—at immorality, at injustice, at ungodly behavior], yet do not sin [wrongdoing]; do not let your anger [cause you shame, nor allow it to] last until the sun goes down. And do not give the devil an opportunity [to lead you into sin by holding a grudge, or nurturing anger, or harboring resentment, or cultivating bitterness]."* (AMP) (sin emphasis pjs)

---

[182] The Edge. (2017) "The Road to Relapse: 8 Dangerous Thoughts to Avoid in Recovery" https://www.theedgerehab.com/blog/relapse-thoughts-to-avoid-in-recovery/

Bitterness is unforgiving! The inability to effectively manage emotions in addiction recovery can lead to significant challenges. Emotional regulation is critical during recovery because substance abuse often serves as a maladaptive coping mechanism for negative emotions. The inability to limit feelings can result in emotional dysregulation, which may increase vulnerability to relapse. Rage is the last refuge of the incompetent!

Dealing with emotions is particularly challenging for many recovering from addiction because they may have used substances to avoid emotional pain. Recovery requires confronting and processing these emotions to heal. Moreover, emotional suppression can lead to an array of problems, including substance abuse, aggression, and psychosomatic illnesses. Emotional escapism, where one avoids dealing with negative emotions, can also lead to a numbing of positive emotions like joy and happiness, which are crucial for a fulfilling life in recovery.

To provide you with the most comprehensive information, I will continue to search for additional sources that offer insight into the difficulties of managing emotions in addiction recovery.

The inability to limit emotions in addiction recovery presents a considerable obstacle, as managing emotions is crucial for maintaining sobriety. Emotional dysregulation can lead to negative behaviors and poor choices, reinforcing the cycle of addiction. In recovery, individuals often experience a wide range of emotions, such as fear, joy, anger, excitement, guilt, worry, boredom, and loneliness. These emotions can become overwhelming, particularly for those who have spent years avoiding their feelings or are out of practice managing them (Mosel, 2023; Kober, 2014).[183] [184]

Acknowledging emotions is the first step in managing them. Suppressing or denying feelings is counterproductive; instead, it is necessary to recognize and address them directly. During recovery,

---

[183] Mosul, S. (2023). "Depression, Anger, and Addiction: The Role of Emotions in Recovery and Treatment" https://americanaddictioncenters.org/co-occurring-disorders/emotions-in-recovery-and-treatment#

[184] Kober, H. (2014). Emotion regulation in substance use disorders. In J. J. Gross (Ed.), Handbook of emotion regulation (p. 428–446). New York: Guilford Press.

withdrawal symptoms can exacerbate emotional instability, making it even more essential to develop effective coping strategies. Implementing self-soothing techniques like deep breathing, grounding exercises, and engaging in positive activities can provide constructive outlets for emotional expression and help stabilize one's emotional state (Covenant, 2023).[185]

Additionally, as recovery progresses, the fluctuating emotional landscape requires individuals to adapt their coping strategies to maintain emotional equilibrium continuously. Ensuring that individuals have access to resources and support for managing emotions is an integral part of a comprehensive recovery program. This support can come in therapy, peer support groups or self-help strategies emphasizing the importance of emotional awareness and regulation.

The Trouble with the Inability to Limit Impulses in Addiction Recovery

Galatians 5:22-23 lists the fruit of the Spirit, which includes self-control. The implication is that a life led by the Spirit should demonstrate control over impulsive actions, which is often compromised in addiction. *"But the fruit of the Spirit [the result of His presence within us] is love [unselfish concern for others], joy, [inner] peace, patience [not the ability to wait, but how we act while waiting], kindness, goodness, faithfulness, gentleness, self-control. Against such things there is no law."* (AMP)

Increased impulsivity leads to a sleepy brain. The trouble with the inability to limit impulses in addiction recovery is linked to the diminished capacity for impulse control often found in individuals with long-standing addictions. This issue is significant because impulse control is closely related to the risk of relapse. The prefrontal cortex, responsible for self-control, becomes less connected with the limbic system, which responds to substance use, making it physically challenging to control impulses.

---

[185] Covenant Hills Treatment Center. (2023) "7 Ways to Manage Emotions and Recovery Successfully After Addiction Treatment" https://covenanthillstreatment. com/managing-emotions-during-addiction/#:~:text=1,and you shouldn't suppress them

Impulse control can be improved through various strategies, including addressing underlying mental health issues, being cautious about social influences, understanding personal triggers, managing one's environment to reduce temptations, and practicing mindfulness to strengthen the prefrontal cortex. Such strategies can help rebuild the connections between brain areas responsible for impulse control, which is crucial for sustained recovery (Recovery 2019).[186] Great things are not done by impulse!

The Trouble with the Inability to Limit Lying in Addiction Recovery

Proverbs 12:22 tells us that the LORD detests lying lips but delights in those who tell the truth. Deceit can be a symptom of deeper issues in the struggle against addiction, indicating a deviation from the path of recovery. *"Lying lips are extremely disgusting to the Lord, But those who deal faithfully are His delight."* (AMP)

The devil was a liar from the beginning! The issue with the difficulty in controlling dishonesty during the process of recovering from addiction is strongly connected to pathological lying, which can arise as a result of or coexist alongside substance/behavioral addiction. A person who consistently lies is not considered mentally ill solely due to this behavior, as it is usually a symptom of other mental health disorders. However, if excessive lying leads to significant problems in one's personal or professional life, seeking professional assistance may be necessary.

Dishonesty wrinkles life! Pathological lying can harm all aspects of an individual's life, including personal and professional relationships. Often stemming from low self-esteem or a distorted self-image, individuals may lie to project an image of trustworthiness or to present themselves as someone they aspire to be.

Individuals who frequently or compulsively lie are categorized as pathological liars. There are two common types of pathological lying:

---

[186] Recovery Ways. (2019) "How Can You Control Your Impulses in Addiction Recovery?" https://www.recoveryways.com/rehab-blog/how-can-you-control-your-impulses-in-addiction-recovery/

mythomania and pseudologia fantastica. Mental health disorders can potentially contribute to this behavior. Obtaining a diagnosis can serve as a starting point in addressing chronic lying. If pathological lying appears to be a harmless annoyance, it may indicate a larger underlying issue. Lying can be an indication of mental health concerns as well as substance abuse. Seeking assistance for mental health issues, including conditions that may lead to pathological lying, is crucial.

This behavior can manifest as a result of various mental health conditions and may require a combination of psychotherapy and medication for effective management. However, treating pathological lying can be complex, as these individuals may even lie to their therapists, making it a challenging disorder to address. Neglecting treatment for pathological lying can result in negative consequences such as social isolation, financial difficulties, and more severe mental health issues like depression (Gallik 2023).[187]

In the recovery journey, individuals may persist in telling falsehoods to evade judgment or shame, perhaps because it is a lingering residue of their previous behaviors. It is of paramount importance to address this matter with compassion and empathy, acknowledging that deception can be indicative of the underlying addictive disorder. As a crucial component of the recovery process, honesty must be upheld and regarded as a vital virtue, drawing inspiration from biblical teachings that emphasize the power of truth. By guiding individuals towards embracing openness, we can provide the support and understanding needed to motivate and inspire their continued progress.

The Trouble with Devaluation of Thoughts in Addiction Recovery

Your conscience is a measure of your selfishness! In Romans 12:2, believers are encouraged not to conform to the pattern of this world but to be transformed by renewing their minds. When someone devalues

---

[187] Gallik, S. (2023) "Pathological Lying: The Dark Side Of Addiction" https://stevegallik.org/pathological-lying-the-dark-side-of-addiction/

their thoughts or beliefs, they may be at risk of relapse by conforming to old patterns of addictive behavior. *"And do not be conformed to this world [any longer with its superficial values and customs] [destructive methods of selfishness], but be transformed and progressively changed [as you mature spiritually] by the renewing of your mind [focusing on godly values and ethical attitudes], so that you may prove [for yourselves] what the will of God is, that which is good and acceptable and perfect [in His plan and purpose for you]."* (AMP) (selfishness emphasis pjs)

In addiction recovery, the devaluation of thoughts can present a significant challenge. Devaluing thoughts are often negative, making it difficult for individuals to have a positive self-perception. Identifying these thoughts and employing positive self-talk and healthy coping mechanisms to combat them is crucial. By doing so, individuals can enhance their self-worth and improve their chances of long-term recovery.

The devaluation of thoughts in addiction recovery is closely linked with cognitive distortions, which are inaccurate thoughts that reinforce negative thinking and emotions. These distortions encompass control fallacies, blaming, "should" statements, emotional reasoning, and more. Such patterns can significantly impact an individual's recovery journey by influencing their self-esteem, emotional well-being, and behavior.

Your actions reveal your thoughts! Cognitive Behavioral Therapy (CBT) and a Bible-based counseling model of right and wrong thinking have proven practical approaches to counteract these cognitive distortions. These methods help individuals reframe their negative thoughts into more rational and positive ones, enhancing recovery and reducing the risk of relapse. Through insightful and motivating references, these approaches provide valuable guidance, inspire change, and offer an uplifting truth (Kessler 2020).[188]

Recognizing cognitive distortions is of the utmost importance as they can discreetly impact our emotions and beliefs, often escaping our awareness until revealed by others. Collaborating with mental health

---

[188] Kessler, C. (2020) "What Are Cognitive Distortions & How They Impact Addiction Recovery" https://lighthouserecoveryinstitute.com/negative-thinking-patterns-in-recovery/

experts to detect and modify these patterns is crucial, paving the way for lasting sobriety and a fulfilling existence.

A darker self-perspective distorts reality. For individuals on the path of addiction recovery, it becomes paramount to acknowledge and confront these cognitive distortions, actively participating in therapeutic interventions aimed at rectifying them. Embracing this life-saving aspect of the recovery journey can genuinely make a transformative difference.

The Bible Says...

(2 Corinthians 10:3-6 REM) — *"Remember that even though we live in the world, the war in which we are engaged is not like wars the world fights. We don't use worldly weapons designed to kill the body or destroy physical structures, nor do we use the world's weapons of lies, distortion, manipulation, deceit, flattery, coercion, sanctions, or trickery. On the contrary, our weapons are from God and have divine power to free the mind, heal the heart, and demolish Satan's stronghold of fear, lies and selfishness. We demolish every idea, argument, doctrine, teaching or concept that infects the mind and distorts or obstructs the truth about God, and we reclaim the thoughts, feelings and attitudes into the truth about God as revealed by Jesus Christ. We stand ready to bring discipline to bear to help break destructive habits so that maturity and health will be fully realized."*

CHAPTER 24

OPTION REDUCTION

The Perils of Option Reduction — Paranoia, Escape, and Out of Control

Addiction recovery can be a challenging journey, fraught with both physical and emotional obstacles. One of the most concerning warning signs of potential relapse is the presence of paranoia, wherein individuals may become excessively suspicious or fearful in their interactions with others. Another troublesome indicator is the need to escape from reality through unhealthy behaviors or substances. This desire to numb oneself can quickly spiral out of control, leading to overwhelming feelings of powerlessness and helplessness. Furthermore, stress and isolation can exacerbate these issues, eventually causing emotional dysregulation. In moments like these, individuals must seek support and guidance from their loved ones and professionals, relying on the truth and inspiration found within the Bible to navigate the path to recovery with renewed hope and strength.

Option Reduction

When nearing addiction relapse, how does the addict perceive their loss of options? When an individual approaching addiction relapse perceives their loss of options, it typically involves a complex interplay of mental, emotional, and situational factors. The perception of diminished choices can be understood from several perspectives (Marlatt 2005).[189]

Addicts often experience *Cognitive Distortions*, where their thinking patterns become skewed. These may include all-or-nothing thinking, overgeneralization, and catastrophizing. They might perceive situations as hopeless or feel they have no control over their circumstances, leading to limited options.

Emotional Dysregulation plays a significant role. Feelings of despair, anxiety, or overwhelming stress can cloud judgment and make it difficult to see alternative courses of action. The intense craving for the substance can override other emotional responses, narrowing their focus to immediate relief rather than long-term well-being.

- **Lack of Emotional Awareness**: Difficulty in recognizing and understanding one's own emotions.
- **Impulse Control Difficulties**: Acting impulsively without considering consequences, often driven by intense emotions.
- **Inability to Use Strategies for Modulating Emotions**: Difficulty employing strategies to soothe oneself or regulate emotional responses in challenging situations.

External Factors like social environment, *stress*, and exposure to cues associated with previous substance use can trigger a relapse. In such contexts, the individual may feel that returning to substance use is the only way to cope or escape.

Learned Helplessness is when individuals feel powerless to change their situation due to past failures. This feeling can be prevalent in addicts who have attempted recovery multiple times. They might perceive relapse as inevitable, reducing their motivation to seek alternatives.

Addiction alters *Neurobiological Factors* such as brain chemistry, affecting decision-making and impulse control. The brain's reward system becomes wired to prioritize substance use, making it challenging to consider other options.

---

[189] Marlatt, G. A., & Donovan, D. M. (Eds.). (2005). Relapse prevention: Maintenance strategies in the treatment of addictive behaviors. Guilford Press.

A perceived or actual *Lack of Support* from family, friends, or healthcare professionals can lead to a feeling of isolation and limited choices. Additionally, lack of access to effective treatment or recovery resources can contribute to this perception.

Addressing this perception requires focusing on strategies to broaden the individual's perspective and reinforce their sense of control and ability to make different choices. This includes Cognitive-behavioral Therapy (CBT) (Beck 1993) or Transformation Prayer Ministry (TPM) (Smith 2018) to address distorted thinking patterns, build emotional resilience, enhance social support, and address neurobiological factors through appropriate medical interventions.[190] [191]

Understanding and addressing these perceptions is critical in preventing relapse and promoting long-term recovery. Addiction is not just a physical dependence but also a psychological and emotional condition that requires a comprehensive approach for effective management.

We will focus on three primary areas that I consider problematic in the reducing options perceived by the one nearing relapse: paranoia, escape, and out-of-control.

Paranoia —When nearing addiction relapse, how does paranoia play out among the loss of options?

Paranoia involves an exaggerated or unfounded mistrust and suspicion towards other individuals, often characterized by a pervasive feeling of being persecuted or targeted. When these feelings of paranoia reach extreme levels, they could indicate the presence of a mental health disorder. This condition is marked not only by its intensity but also by its detachment from reality, where the individual's perceptions and beliefs about others' intentions towards them are skewed despite a lack of concrete evidence. In clinical settings, such extreme manifestations

---

[190] Beck, A. T., Wright, F. D., Newman, C. F., & Liese, B. S. (1993). *Cognitive therapy of substance abuse.* Guilford Press.

[191] Smith, E., Smith, J. (2018) "Effortless Forgiveness." New Creation Publishing, Campbellsville, KY.

of paranoia are carefully evaluated, as they can be symptomatic of various psychological conditions, including paranoid personality disorder, schizophrenia, or delusional disorder. Identifying and treating such situations is vital for the mental and emotional well-being of the individual.

Aggravation of Pre-Existing Mental Health Conditions: Many individuals with substance use disorders also have co-occurring mental health conditions, such as anxiety disorders or schizophrenia, where paranoia is a key symptom. Substance use can exacerbate these conditions, leading to heightened paranoia. This can create a distorted perception of reality, causing individuals to feel that they are trapped or have no alternatives other than returning to substance use (Drake 2007).[192]

Substance-Induced Paranoia: Certain substances, especially stimulants like cocaine and methamphetamine, can induce paranoia in users. This drug-induced paranoia can cause mistrust and suspicion, making individuals feel isolated and unsupported, which might narrow their perceived options for coping or seeking help (Mahoney 2015).[193]

Impact on Decision-Making and Problem-Solving: Paranoia can impair decision-making and problem-solving abilities. In the context of addiction and relapse, this impairment can lead to a reduced capacity to evaluate situations realistically, consider the long-term consequences of their actions, or identify and utilize available support and treatment options (Verdejo-Garcia 2007).[194]

Social Isolation and Loss of Support: Paranoia often leads to social withdrawal and isolation. In the context of addiction recovery, this can result in the loss of social support, which is a crucial factor in

[192] Drake, R. E., Mueser, K. T., & Brunette, M. F. (2007). Management of persons with co-occurring severe mental illness and substance use disorder: Program implications. *World Psychiatry, 6*(3), 131–136.

[193] Mahoney III, J. J., Thompson-Lake, D. G., Cooper, K., Verrico, C. D., Newton, T. F., & De La Garza II, R. (2015). A comparison of impulsivity and sensation seeking in cocaine users and healthy controls. *Drug and Alcohol Dependence, 149*, 293-298.

[194] Verdejo-Garcia, A., Bechara, A., Recknor, E. C., & Pérez-García, M. (2007). Negative emotion-driven impulsivity predicts substance dependence problems. *Drug and Alcohol Dependence, 91*(2-3), 213-219.

preventing relapse. The individual may feel that they cannot trust their support network or that others are conspiring against them, making them feel alone in their struggle (Tracy 2016).[195]

Understanding and addressing paranoia in the context of addiction recovery is crucial. Treatment approaches should be holistic, addressing both the substance use disorder and any underlying or co-occurring mental health conditions. This might include a combination of pharmacotherapy, cognitive-behavioral therapy, and supportive therapies to build social skills and coping mechanisms.

Escape —How does escape play out among the loss of options?

The concept of *Escape* plays a significant role in the dynamics of addiction relapse, particularly in the context of perceived loss of options. This can be understood through various mental, emotional, and behavioral aspects.

Escape as a Coping Mechanism: For many individuals with addiction, substance use is a means to escape from negative emotions, stress, or traumatic experiences. When faced with challenges or discomfort, the perceived lack of options can lead to relapse as an escape route. This is often reinforced by previous patterns where substance use provided temporary relief from psychological distress (Khantzian 1997).[196]

Cognitive Escape and Avoidance: In the face of stress or triggers, individuals may engage in mental escape, where they avoid thinking about the consequences of their actions or the possibilities of coping without substances. This avoidance can contribute to a narrowed perception of available options, making relapse seem like the only viable alternative (Marlatt 1985).[197]

---

[195] Tracy, K., & Wallace, S. P. (2016). Benefits of peer support groups in the treatment of addiction. *Substance Abuse and Rehabilitation, 7*, 143–154.

[196] Khantzian, E. J. (1997). The self-medication hypothesis of substance use disorders: A reconsideration and recent applications. *Harvard Review of Psychiatry, 4*(5), 231-244.

[197] Marlatt, G. A., & Gordon, J. R. (1985). Relapse prevention: Maintenance strategies in the treatment of addictive behaviors. Guilford Press.

Behavioral and Emotional Escape: As pressures and negative emotions build up, the individual might seek an immediate escape, which often manifests as relapse. This is particularly true in cases where the individual lacks healthy coping mechanisms or support systems (Witkiewitz 2004).[198]

Environmental and Social Influences: The environment and social context can play a role in escape-seeking behaviors. For example, being in a setting where substances are readily available or being around others who use them can increase the temptation to use substances as an escape (Moos 2006).[199]

In addressing the role of escape in the context of addiction relapse, therapeutic interventions should focus on developing healthier coping mechanisms, addressing underlying emotional and psychological issues, and building a supportive environment that reduces the need for escape through substance use. Cognitive-behavioral therapy, mindfulness-based interventions, and supportive counseling can be particularly effective.

Out of Control —How does feeling out of control play out among the loss of options?

When an individual nearing addiction relapse feels out of control, this sensation significantly influences their perception of options and decision-making processes. This phenomenon is multifaceted and deeply rooted in both the mental and emotional underpinnings of addiction and the nature of relapse itself.

Loss of Control and Impaired Decision-Making: Feeling out of control is often linked with impaired decision-making abilities. For someone with a history of addiction, this can lead to a narrowed perception of choices, where substance use appears as the only or

---

[198] Witkiewitz, K., & Marlatt, G. A. (2004). Relapse prevention for alcohol and drug problems: That was Zen, this is Tao. *American Psychologist, 59*(4), 224-235.

[199] Moos, R. H., & Moos, B. S. (2006). Rates and predictors of relapse after natural and treated remission from alcohol use disorders. *Addiction, 101*(2), 212-222.

most accessible option to regain a sense of control or alleviate distress (Bechara 2002).[200]

Role of Executive Function in Addiction Relapse: Executive functions, which include planning, impulse control, and foreseeing the consequences of actions, are often compromised in addiction. The Addictive Personality located in the Brain's Limbic System is drawing a higher rate of metabolic flow than the "upper-room," higher thinking region (top half of the brain). When an individual feels out of control, these functions may be further impaired, limiting their ability to see and evaluate the full range of options (Goldstein 2002).[201]

Emotional Dysregulation and Relapse: Emotional dysregulation is a common challenge among individuals with substance use disorders. The inability to control emotions is a common sign of Addictive Personality control. When overwhelmed by feelings and feeling out of control, the individual may revert to familiar patterns of substance use as a maladaptive coping mechanism, perceiving few or no alternatives (Fox 2007).[202]

Stress-Induced Relapse: High levels of stress, often accompanied by feelings of being out of control, are a significant trigger for relapse. Stress-induced anxiety can impair judgment and the ability to consider long-term consequences, leading to a focus on immediate relief through substance use (Sin 2007).[203]

Social and Environmental Factors: The individual's social and environmental context can exacerbate feelings of losing control. For example, a lack of a supportive network or being in an environment that

---

[200] Bechara, A., & Damasio, H. (2002). Decision-making and addiction (part I): Impaired activation of somatic states in substance dependent individuals when pondering decisions with negative future consequences. *Neuropsychologia, 40*(10), 1675-1689.

[201] Goldstein, R. Z., & Volkow, N. D. (2002). Drug addiction and its underlying neurobiological basis: Neuroimaging evidence for the involvement of the frontal cortex. *American Journal of Psychiatry, 159*(10), 1642-1652.

[202] Fox, H. C., Axelrod, S. R., Paliwal, P., Sleeper, J., & Sinha, R. (2007). Difficulties in emotion regulation and impulse control during cocaine abstinence. *Drug and Alcohol Dependence, 89*(2-3), 298-301.

[203] Sinha, R. (2007). The role of stress in addiction relapse. *Current Psychiatry Reports, 9*(5), 388-395.

triggers memories of substance use can increase the sense of helplessness and narrow perceived options (Moos 2006).[204]

Addressing the feeling of being out of control in the context of addiction relapse involves a comprehensive approach. This includes enhancing coping skills, improving stress management, strengthening executive functions through cognitive rehabilitation, and creating a supportive environment. Counseling interventions like cognitive-behavioral therapy, transformation prayer ministry, mindfulness practices, and relapse prevention strategies are crucial.

At this critical moment, we are calling the "Option Reduction," my thoughts naturally gravitate toward the poignant episode of Jesus Christ in the Garden of Gethsemane. This instance stands out as it marks one of the rare occasions where Jesus openly expressed a sense of profound distress with overwhelming thoughts and feelings.

This significant event, unfolding just before His arrest, trial, and eventual crucifixion, is vividly captured in the Gospel of Matthew 26:36-46 (NIV). The scripture recounts how Jesus, engulfed in deep sorrow, confided in His disciples, *"My soul is overwhelmed with sorrow to the point of death."* He implored them to remain vigilant while He sought consolation through prayer, ultimately prostrating Himself in earnest supplication.

This narrative offers profound insights, especially when considering how we, too, may find ourselves overwhelmed by life's daunting challenges. There are three key lessons to be gleaned from Jesus' response in this moment of turmoil. **First** and foremost, Jesus exemplified absolute candor in acknowledging His emotional state. His willingness to be vulnerable and transparent about His feelings is a lesson in emotional honesty. **Secondly**, He demonstrated the importance of seeking support, as He enlisted the companionship and vigilance of His closest friends during this trying time. **Lastly**, Jesus turned to prayer, laying His burdens before His Father, underscoring the power of spiritual communion in times of distress.

These actions of Jesus serve as an exemplary model for us,

---

[204] Moos, R. H., & Moos, B. S. (2006). Rates and predictors of relapse after natural and treated remission from alcohol use disorders. *Addiction, 101*(2), 212-222.

especially when faced with overwhelming circumstances. They teach us the value of honesty in confronting our emotions, the significance of seeking support from those around us, and the transformative power of prayer in navigating life's trials. This holistic approach, encompassing emotional, social, and spiritual dimensions, provides a comprehensive framework for coping with and overcoming our challenges.

The Bible Says...

(Hebrews 4:14-16 REM) — *"Therefore, since we have a great high priest (a great physician) who has gone through the heavens—Jesus, the Son of God—let us hold confidently to the truth about God and his plan to heal and restore us. For we do not have a heavenly physician (a great high priest) who is unable to appreciate our weakness, suffering and struggles, but we have one who in his humanity was tempted in every way—exactly as we are—yet without sin, without ever giving in to selfish temptations. Therefore, let us approach the throne of God's grace without fear, but confidently, realizing that he longs to dispense all the resources of heaven to heal us so that we may receive mercy, grace, and every benefit to give us victory in our time of need."*

CHAPTER 25

RELAPSE — RETURNING TO USE AND ABUSE

The Perils of Returning to Use and Abuse:
Unveiling the Harsh Reality of Relapse!

John's Unseen Struggle and Illusion of Control

Once, a man named John lived in the bustling city of New York. John had struggled with addiction for many years but had recently celebrated his fifth year of sobriety. The journey hadn't been easy. Every day was a battle against his inner demons, but John felt he had finally gained control over his life. He had a stable job, a loving family, and a support group that kept him grounded.

One evening, John attended a friend's birthday party. The air was filled with laughter, music, and the clinking of glasses. Initially, he felt confident in his ability to resist temptation, but as the night progressed, the atmosphere of festivity started to chip away at his resolve. The sight and smell of alcohol, which he had avoided for years, began to stir something within him.

In a moment of weakness, John convinced himself that one drink wouldn't hurt. He thought he had mastered his addiction and could handle it. However, the moment the liquid touched his lips, years of hard work started to unravel. That one drink turned into two and then more until he lost count. The feeling of euphoria was intoxicating, and he delved deeper into his old habits, forgetting the pain and struggle it had taken to break free from them.

The Harsh Awakening

The following day, John woke up with a throbbing headache, a feeling of deep shame, and the bitter realization that he had relapsed. The guilt was overwhelming. He had let down not only himself but also his family and friends who had stood by him through his journey to sobriety. The reality of addiction relapse hit him hard; it was not just a single moment of weakness but a robust and ongoing battle against a relentless enemy.

The Road to Recovery, Again

John understood the importance of beginning anew and contacted his support circle. He humbly admitted his relapse to them, and they warmly embraced him, recognizing that the journey to recovery is a complex one with both triumphs and setbacks. John took the courageous step of seeking guidance from a Christian counselor, acknowledging that he must not only address the root causes of his relapse but also confront the spiritual aspects he had previously neglected. This decision demonstrates his desire for truth, inspiration, and personal growth along his path to wholeness.

John began a spiritual journey of compassion and understanding, aligning with Christian values of love, forgiveness, and healing. He gained insights into the complexities of addiction, aiding in the development of more effective, empathetic, and holistic treatment, not just the physical but also the mental, emotional, and spiritual dimensions of recovery.

The Lesson Learned

Through this challenging experience, John learned that addiction is a cunning and baffling disease, always lurking in the shadows, waiting for a moment of vulnerability. He understood that sobriety wasn't just about abstaining from substances but also about constant vigilance and self-awareness. He began to work even harder on his recovery, attending meetings and helping others who were struggling with addiction.

A New Hope

As time passed, John's life started to stabilize again. He found new ways to cope with stress and triggers. He became an active member of the recovery community, sharing his story of relapse to help others understand the importance of remaining vigilant. Though he knew the road ahead would always have its challenges, he was now more equipped to face them.

The Unending Journey

John's journey serves as a poignant reminder of the harsh reality of addiction relapse. It's a path that many have walked and will continue to walk. However, it's also a testament to the human spirit's resilience and the power of community and support in overcoming life's toughest challenges.

The phenomenon of relapsing into substance addiction releases a cascade of issues characterized by physical, emotional, and spiritual disintegration. This collapse, often experienced during a return to substance abuse, entails a series of profound and intricate changes.

Physical Collapse in Addiction Relapse — *The Body's Role in Addiction and Relapse!*

Physically, the body, having once adapted to the absence of the substance — neuroadaptation — faces a sudden and often severe shock when the substance is reintroduced. This reintroduction can lead to a range of physiological responses, including heightened tolerance, withdrawal symptoms, and a potential exacerbation of physical health issues. The physical toll is significant, as the body struggles to recalibrate to the presence of the addictive substance once again (Volkow, Koob, & McLellan, 2016).[205]

Relapse can reverse the gains made during detoxification, leading to the re-emergence of withdrawal symptoms. These may include nausea, sweating, shakiness, and, in severe cases, seizures or delirium (American Psychiatric Association, 2013).[206]

Tolerance to substances often decreases during periods of abstinence. If an individual relapses and consumes the same amount of substance as they did previously, this can lead to overdose because the body's threshold for the substance has lowered (Doweiko, 2015).[207]

Emotional Collapse in Addiction Relapse — *Navigating the Mental and Emotional Terrain!*

Emotionally, the relapse into addiction marks a critical setback. It often engenders a deep sense of failure, guilt, and despair, which can intensify the addictive behavior. The emotional turmoil is compounded by the re-emergence of feelings and coping mechanisms the individual had previously tried to overcome. These emotions can stem from perceived personal failure or the disappointment of others (Marlatt & Donovan, 2005).

This can lead to a vicious cycle, where emotional distress fuels further substance use, and the addiction deepens as a means of escape or coping.[208]

Substance abuse is closely linked with mental health disorders. Relapse can worsen symptoms of existing mental health conditions,

[205] Volkow, N. D., Koob, G. F., & McLellan, A. T. (2016). Neurobiologic advances from the brain disease model of addiction. *New England Journal of Medicine, 374*(4), 363-371.

[206] American Psychiatric Association. (2013). Diagnostic and statistical manual of mental disorders (5th ed.). Washington, DC: Author.

[207] Doweiko, H. E. (2015). Concepts of chemical dependency. Cengage Learning.

[208] Marlatt, G. A., & Donovan, D. M. (Eds.). (2005). Relapse prevention: Maintenance strategies in the treatment of addictive behaviors. Guilford Press.

such as depression and anxiety, leading to a deteriorated emotional state (National Institute on Drug Abuse, 2018).[209]

The act of relapsing can foster feelings of hopelessness and despair, as individuals might believe they are unable to overcome their addiction. This emotional state can hinder recovery efforts (Melemis, 2015).[210]

Understanding the dual nature of this collapse — the physical and the emotional — is vital for effective intervention and support. It requires a comprehensive approach that addresses both the physiological aspects of addiction and the mental and emotional factors that contribute to the cycle of abuse and relapse. This dual-focus strategy is crucial for offering holistic care and support, aiming not just at the cessation of substance use but also at the emotional and mental well-being of the individual.

This comprehensive understanding of the physical and emotional collapse associated with addiction relapse is crucial for effective treatment and support, providing a foundation for therapeutic interventions focused on both the physical and emotional aspects of recovery.

In recovery, flawed perspectives, emotional pain, and troublesome behaviors are not the problem. The problem is actually in what they believe. Their perspectives, emotions, and behaviors all reflect their heart's beliefs. Without changing their heart belief of being dirty, tainted, and damaged, they will view hope (God) as distant and unattainable. Their thoughts become the lenses in which they interpret their lives.

Biblical Aspects of Addiction Relapse — *Finding Strength Beyond the Physical and Emotional!*

Understanding the biblical aspects of relapsing into substance addiction involves examining scripture for insights into human weaknesses, the nature of temptation, and the process of healing and redemption. The Bible, while not explicitly discussing substance addiction as understood

---

[209] National Institute on Drug Abuse. (2018). Comorbidity: Substance use disorders and other mental illnesses. Retrieved from https://www.drugabuse.gov/publications/drugfacts/comorbidity-substance-use-disorders-other-mental-illnesses

[210] Melemis, S. M. (2015). Relapse prevention and the five rules of recovery. *Yale Journal of Biology and Medicine, 88*(3), 325.

today, provides principles that can be applied to the struggle against addiction and the experience of relapse (McMinn 2007).[211]

The Bible acknowledges human frailty and susceptibility to temptation — human weakness due to sin. In Romans 7:19, Paul reflects on the struggle with sin: *"For I do not do the good I want to do, but the evil I do not want to do—this I keep on doing"* (NIV). This verse can be interpreted as a recognition of the ongoing struggle against destructive behaviors akin to substance addiction.

Despite acknowledging human weakness, the Bible also offers hope and the possibility of redemption. Isaiah 40:31 (NIV) states, *"But those who hope in the Lord will renew their strength. They will soar on wings like eagles; they will run and not grow weary, they will walk and not be faint."* This passage is often seen as encouragement for those facing relapse, suggesting that renewal and strength are possible through faith.

God's compassionate forgiveness is central to Christian teachings and can be particularly relevant to those who have relapsed. In 1 John 1:9 (NIV), it is written, *"If we confess our sins, He is faithful and just and will forgive us our sins and purify us from all unrighteousness."* This verse speaks to the importance of seeking forgiveness and the availability of God's grace, even after a setback.

The Bible emphasizes the role of community in supporting individuals through challenges. Galatians 6:2 (NIV) instructs, *"Carry each other's burdens, and in this way, you will fulfill the law of Christ."* This suggests the importance of a supportive community in the journey of recovery and the significance of not facing struggles alone.

The theme of perseverance is recurrent in the Bible and can apply to overcoming addiction. James 1:12 (NIV) says, *"Blessed is the one who perseveres under trial because, having stood the test, that person will receive the crown of life that the Lord has promised to those who love Him."* This can be interpreted as encouragement to persist in the face of relapse and continue striving towards recovery.

Ephesians 6:12 (NIV) discusses the concept of spiritual warfare: *"For our struggle is not against flesh and blood, but against the rulers,*

---

[211] McMinn, M. R., & Campbell, C. D. (2007). Integrative Psychotherapy: Toward a Comprehensive Christian Approach. IVP Academic.

against the authorities, against the powers of this dark world and against the spiritual forces of evil in the heavenly realms." This can be understood as an acknowledgment of the spiritual dimensions of struggles like addiction.

While the Bible does not explicitly address substance addiction and relapse in modern terms, its teachings offer insights and principles that can be applied to these challenges. These include recognizing human weakness, the hope of redemption, the importance of forgiveness and community support, and the necessity of perseverance and awareness of spiritual aspects (Johnson 2010).[212]

We Perceive What We Believe

"Yesterday is history, tomorrow is a mystery, today is a gift of God, which is why we call it the present" —Bill Keane.[213]

The addict is seeing whatever they believe because they are viewing life through distorted lenses. Unchanged beliefs will result in a continuation of feeling what they thought during their active addiction lifestyle. Emotional pain is an indicator of a more significant problem involving beliefs. Simply changing thinking about the belief will not dissuade the heart from the idea.

A deep-seated belief in emotional pain and suffering awakens our awareness of pain's power, guides us toward acknowledging its existence, and ignites a solid desire to respond.

We must allow ourselves to feel emotionally damaging pain when we believe lies. When we think truthfully, we must also feel peace, joy, contentment, and other positive emotions. Often, the behavior of addiction is not the problem but the futile attempt to solve the problem. The alcoholic doesn't have a drinking problem. They are drinking to solve a perceived problem. Substance and behavioral abuse

---

[212] Johnson, E. L. (2010). Foundations for Soul Care: A Christian Psychology Proposal. IVP Academic.

[213] Retrieved from https://quotefancy.com/quote/53/Bil-Keane-Yesterday-is-history-tomorrow-is-a-mystery-today-is-a-gift-of-God-which-is-why#:~:text=Bil Keane Quote: "Yesterday is,we call it the present."

are short-sighted attempts to solve perceived problems. Whether it is anxiety, stress, or boredom, recovery relapse is a futile attempt to appease what they are trying to distract themselves from. Simply telling them the truth does not bring remedy due to their flawed perceptions, emotions, and beliefs.

To say the alcoholic doesn't have a drinking problem is a phrase implying the core problem is alcohol consumption itself. Instead, the underlying issues that lead to alcoholism are the actual problem. These can include emotional or mental health issues, trauma, stress, or other psychological factors. Alcohol is seen more as a symptom or a coping mechanism for these more profound problems.

From a Christian counseling perspective, this phrase can be understood as recognizing the need for a holistic approach to treatment. It's not just about stopping the use and abuse but also about addressing the spiritual, mental, and emotional needs of the individual. The focus is on healing the whole person — spirit, soul, and body.

Understanding the Complexity of Relapse

Relapse is not just a singular event but a process that unfolds over time, marked by a return to substance abuse. This process is often triggered by various factors, which can be emotional, physical, or environmental. Understanding these triggers is crucial in developing effective strategies for prevention and management.

The physical dimension of relapse involves the body's conditioned response to substances. This biological aspect underscores the importance of medical and therapeutic interventions in treating substance addiction. Medications, along with therapies like cognitive-behavioral therapy, can play a pivotal role in mitigating the physical cravings and withdrawal symptoms that often lead to relapse.

Emotional triggers, such as stress, anxiety, or depression, are significant contributors to relapse. It's vital to address these underlying emotional issues through counseling, support groups, and personal development. Developing coping mechanisms and emotional resilience is key to preventing relapse.

The spiritual aspect of relapse and recovery often involves a journey of self-discovery and meaning-making. Many find strength and motivation in their faith, spiritual beliefs, or connection to something greater than themselves. This spiritual grounding can provide the resilience and perspective needed to overcome the challenges of addiction and relapse.

An integrative approach that combines physical, emotional, and spiritual strategies offers the best chance for successful recovery and prevention of relapse. Tailored treatment plans that address the individual's unique needs and circumstances are essential.

Educating individuals about the nature of addiction and the process of recovery empowers them to take active roles in their healing journey. Support from family, friends, and recovery communities is invaluable in providing the encouragement and accountability necessary for sustained recovery.

Finally, it is crucial to emphasize that relapse, while a setback, is not the end of the road. It can be a part of the learning process in the journey towards recovery. With the proper support, tools, and mindset, individuals struggling with substance addiction can find their path to a healthier, substance-free life.

The Bible Says...

(Romans 7:14-25 REM) — *"We know that the law is consistent, reliable and reasonable; but I am inconsistent, unreliable and unreasonable, because the infection of distrust, fear and selfishness has warped my mind and damaged my thinking. I am frustrated with what I do! For having been restored to trust, I want to do what is in harmony with God and his methods and principles; but I find that even though I trust God, my old habits, conditioned responses, preconceived ideas and other remnants of the devastation caused by distrust and selfishness are not yet fully removed. And if I find an old habit causing me to behave in ways that I now find detestable, I affirm that the law is a very helpful tool revealing residual damage in need of healing. What is happening is this: I have come to trust God, and I desire to do his will, but old habits and conditioned responses*

— which present almost reflexively in certain situations — have not yet been totally eliminated and thus cause me to do things I do not want to do. I know that my mind was completely infected with distrust, fear and selfishness, which totally perverted all my desires and faculties, so that even when distrust has been eradicated and trust has been restored, the damage caused by years of distrustful and selfish behavior has not yet been fully healed. So, I find that at times, I have the desire to do what is right, but do not yet have the ability to carry out the desire. For the old habits and conditioned responses are not the good I want to do: No! They are remnants of my selfish, unconverted mind. So, if I find myself doing what I no longer desire to do, it is not myself that acts, but the vestiges of old habits and conditioned responses that have yet to be removed. And through God's grace, they will soon be removed. So I find this reality at work: When I want to do good, my old selfish habits and residual feelings of fear are right there with me. In my mind, I rejoice in God's methods and principles, but I recognize that I remain damaged from years of being infected with distrust and practicing Satan's methods, so that even though the infection of distrust has been removed, the old habits of fear and self-promotion tempt me from within. What a damaged and corrupt man I am! Who will deliver and heal me from a brain and body so diseased and deformed? Praise be to God—for he has provided the healing solution through Jesus Christ our Lord! So then, I find that in my mind I am now renewed with trust in God and love of his methods, but my brain and body remain damaged by years of self-indulgent behavior." (Bible Scripture Paraphrase)

CHAPTER 26

RETHINKING RECOVERY —
A CLOSER LOOK AT THE 28-DAY
ADDICTION TREATMENT MODEL!

In the ever-evolving landscape of addiction treatment, the pursuit of effective strategies remains paramount. Recent studies shed light on a stark reality: the widely adopted 28-day addiction treatment program, long considered a cornerstone in the fight against addiction, might not be as effective as once thought. These revelations compel us to reassess our approaches and seek better solutions.

The statistics are sobering. Current research indicates that the success rate of these month-long programs hovers around the 20% mark. This figure not only highlights the complexity and tenacity of addiction as a multifaceted health issue but also underscores the necessity for continuous innovation in treatment methodologies.

The 28-day model, rooted in historical practices rather than empirical evidence, has dominated the addiction treatment landscape for decades. Initially, it was shaped by practical considerations, such as insurance policy structures and societal norms, rather than a deep understanding of addiction's nature. The emerging data now invites us to question and reconceptualize this traditional model.

In this blog, we will delve into the intricacies of the 28-day addiction treatment program. We will explore its origins, evaluate its strengths and shortcomings based on the latest research, and discuss alternative approaches that promise greater efficacy. Our journey will take us through a comprehensive examination of what addiction recovery looks like in the modern era, keeping in mind the goal of achieving not just sobriety but holistic healing and long-term wellness.

Join us as we navigate these revelations, seeking clarity, insight, and effective remedies to pursue a more successful path to addiction recovery. Together, we will explore how these findings can catalyze change, drive innovation, and lead to more effective and compassionate addiction treatment strategies.

Intricacies of a 28-day Addiction Treatment

Delving into a 28-day addiction treatment program's structure, methods, and goals can help one understand its intricacies. This program's framework is typically grounded in a multifaceted approach, which may include medical, mental, emotional, and holistic methods tailored to address the complexities of addiction. It's important to note that while I provide a general overview, the specifics can vary based on the institution and the patient's individual needs.

Structure of the 28-Day Program

Assessment and Detoxification —The program often begins with a thorough assessment of the patient's physical and mental health, followed by a medically supervised detoxification process. This phase is critical as it manages withdrawal symptoms in a safe environment (ASAM, 2020).[214]

Individual Therapy — Individual counseling sessions are a cornerstone of the program, where cognitive-behavioral therapy (CBT) and other therapeutic—healing — approaches are employed

---

[214] ASAM. American Society of Addiction Medicine. (2020). National practice guideline for the treatment of opioid use disorder.

to address underlying issues contributing to addiction (McHugh et al., 2010).[215]

Group Therapy — Group sessions provide peer support and facilitate sharing experiences, enhancing social skills and fostering community (Kelly et al., 2011).[216]

Educational Workshops — These workshops educate patients about the nature of addiction, relapse prevention strategies, and healthy coping mechanisms (Melemis, 2015).[217]

Family Therapy — Family involvement can be critical, providing a support system for the patient and addressing any familial issues that may contribute to the addictive behavior (O'Farrell & Fals-Stewart, 2006).[218]

Aftercare Planning — Towards the end of the program, aftercare planning becomes a focus to ensure the patient has a support system and resources for continued recovery post-treatment (McLellan et al., 2000).[219]

Goals and Outcomes

The overarching aim of our therapeutic approach is to assist individuals in attaining and sustaining a state of sobriety. This goal is not just about abstaining from substances but involves a comprehensive transformation of one's lifestyle. Key to this process is developing and

---

[215] McHugh, R. K., Hearon, B. A., & Otto, M. W. (2010). Cognitive-behavioral therapy for substance use disorders. *Psychiatric Clinics of North America, 33*(3), 511-525.

[216] Kelly, J. F., Stout, R. L., Magill, M., Tonigan, J. S., & Pagano, M. E. (2011). The role of Alcoholics Anonymous in mobilizing adaptive social network changes: A prospective lagged mediational analysis. *Drug and Alcohol Dependence, 114*(2-3), 119-126.

[217] Melemis, S. M. (2015). Relapse Prevention and the Five Rules of Recovery. *The Yale Journal of Biology and Medicine, 88*(3), 325–332.

[218] O'Farrell, T. J., & Fals-Stewart, W. (2006). Behavioral couples therapy for alcoholism and drug abuse. *Journal of Substance Abuse Treatment, 30*(2), 113-121.

[219] McLellan, A. T., Lewis, D. C., O'Brien, C. P., & Kleber, H. D. (2000). Drug dependence, a chronic medical illness: implications for treatment, insurance, and outcomes evaluation. *Journal of the American Medical Association, 284*(13), 1689-1695.

enhancing coping strategies that enable individuals to manage potential triggers and avert the risk of relapse effectively. Such skills are critical in navigating the complexities of addiction and recovery.

Moreover, in the more successful programs, there is a significant emphasis on improving spiritual, mental, emotional, and physical health. Substance abuse often takes a considerable toll on an individual's overall well-being. Thus, our therapeutic — healing — interventions are designed to address these multifaceted health concerns, nurturing a holistic recovery process.

Additionally, quality programs recognize the profound impact that substance abuse can have on personal and professional relationships. A well-rounded program places a strong emphasis on the repair and reconstruction of these relationships. Through various therapeutic modalities, treatment facilitates the process of healing and reconciliation, aiding patients in mending the bonds that have been strained or broken due to their struggles with addiction.

Lastly, the more successful treatment programs encourage and support a fundamental shift in lifestyle, steering towards healthier habits. This encompasses physical health through diet, exercise, and spiritual, mental, and emotional well-being. By fostering such changes, these programs aim to lay a foundation for long-term recovery, significantly reducing the likelihood of relapse.

This holistic approach, grounded in evidence-based practices, is instrumental in guiding individuals toward recovery and wellness. The journey toward sobriety involves many layers, requiring a comprehensive strategy that addresses the physical, mental, emotional, and spiritual aspects of healing.

Critiques and Considerations

The efficacy of specific interventions is notably subject to variation, contingent upon individuals' specific conditions and backgrounds. This variability underscores the limitation of standardized methodologies, prompting experts to recommend more tailored strategies for effective outcomes.

Simpson (2004) critically examines the pitfalls of a generalized approach in therapeutic settings, arguing that it fails to accommodate individuals' diverse needs and situations. He advocates for the necessity of customizing treatment plans to enhance their effectiveness.[220]

Similarly, the debate regarding the adequacy of treatment duration remains contentious. The National Institute on Drug Abuse (NIDA) in 2018 highlighted this issue, with proponents of extended treatment durations emphasizing their potential for engendering more profound and enduring transformations in patients. These discussions point towards a growing consensus in the medical and psychological communities about the need for flexible and individualized treatment modalities.[221]

Exploring the Origins

The origins of the 28-day addiction treatment program can be traced back to several historical and medical factors. I will explore the historical context, medical models' influence, and addiction treatment evolution to provide a comprehensive understanding.

Historical Context and Development

The 28-day program is closely linked to the Minnesota Model, developed in the 1950s. This model, originating at the Hazelden Foundation (now Hazelden Betty Ford Foundation) and Willmar State Hospital in Minnesota, was one of the first to treat alcoholism as a disease rather than a moral failing. This approach emphasized a multidisciplinary treatment plan involving doctors, nurses, psychologists, and other professionals.[222]

---

[220] Simpson, D. D. (2004). A conceptual framework for drug treatment process and outcomes. Journal of Substance Abuse Treatment, 27(2), 99-121.

[221] National Institute on Drug Abuse. (2018). Principles of Drug Addiction Treatment: A Research-Based Guide (Third Edition). Retrieved from https://www.drugabuse.gov/publications/principles-drug-addiction-treatment-research-based-guide-third-edition

[222] "The History of the Minnesota Model." Hazelden Betty Ford Foundation. Hazelden Betty Ford Foundation.

The U.S. Armed Forces, recognizing the effectiveness of the Minnesota Model, adopted a similar approach for treating substance abuse among service members. This further legitimized and standardized the 28-day duration as a framework for treatment programs.

Medical and Psychosocial Factors

The 28 days were considered optimal for allowing a safe detoxification process and providing enough time for physical stabilization. The first week typically focuses on managing withdrawal symptoms, followed by intensive therapy in the subsequent weeks.[223]

The program allocates time for patients to learn about addiction, develop coping strategies, and begin the process of behavior change. This period was considered long enough to establish new habits while being short enough to be feasible for most patients to commit.

Development and Critique

Practical considerations, including insurance reimbursement policies also influenced the duration of these programs. Initially, insurance companies were more willing to cover a fixed, short-term stay in a treatment facility, making the 28-day model financially viable.

Over time, the effectiveness of the 28-day model has been questioned. Critics argue that addiction is a chronic condition and requires long-term treatment and support. This has led to the development of extended care programs, outpatient services, and ongoing support groups to supplement the short-term inpatient model.[224]

While the 28-day addiction treatment program has its roots in the mid-20th century with the Minnesota Model, it has evolved.

---

[223] McLellan, A. T., Lewis, D. C., O'Brien, C. P., & Kleber, H. D. (2000). Drug dependence, a chronic medical illness: Implications for treatment, insurance, and outcomes evaluation. JAMA, 284(13), 1689-1695.

[224] White, W. L. (1998). Slaying the Dragon: The History of Addiction Treatment and Recovery in America. Bloomington, IL: Chestnut Health Systems.

The model reflects a balance between medical, psychological, and practical considerations. However, as an understanding of addiction has deepened, the treatment approaches have become more diversified, focusing on long-term care and personalized treatment plans.

Evaluating the 28-day Model

The evaluation of the 28-day addiction treatment model, often termed the "Minnesota Model," is an intricate topic composed of numerous aspects. This model has been a cornerstone in addiction treatment for many decades, yet it is continuously scrutinized and evaluated in light of new research and emerging treatment methodologies. Let's explore the strengths and shortcomings of this model based on recent studies and expert opinions.

Strengths of the 28-Day Addiction Treatment Model

The 28-day model provides a highly structured environment, which can benefit individuals in the early stages of recovery. It offers a routine that includes therapy, support groups, and other therapeutic activities, which can help establish a foundation for long-term sobriety (McKay, J. R., 2009).[225]

This model emphasizes abstinence from addictive substances, which is a crucial step in the recovery process. It provides a safe space away from potential triggers and opportunities to use substances (Simpson & Joe, 2004).[226]

Patients are introduced to support networks such as Alcoholics Anonymous (AA) or Narcotics Anonymous (NA). This exposure can

---

[225] McKay, J. R. (2009). Continuing Care Research: What We Have Learned and Where We Are Going. *Journal of Substance Abuse Treatment*, 36(2), 131–145. https://doi.org/10.1016/j.jsat.2008.10.004

[226] Simpson, D. D., & Joe, G. W. (2004). A longitudinal evaluation of treatment engagement and recovery stages. *Journal of Substance Abuse Treatment*, 27(2), 89–97. https://doi.org/10.1016/j.jsat.2004.06.001

be instrumental in building a community-based support system for post-treatment recovery (Kelly & Yeterian, 2011).[227]

Many 28-day programs incorporate a holistic approach, addressing not only the addiction but also underlying mental, emotional, social, and spiritual factors. This comprehensive care can be crucial in treating the root causes of addiction (Polcin & Henderson, 2008).[228]

Shortcomings of the 28-Day Addiction Treatment Model

Critics argue that the 28-day model adopts a one-size-fits-all approach, which may only be suitable for some individuals or types of addiction. Personalized treatment plans based on individual needs can be more effective (McLellan, A. T., et al., 2005).[229]

The duration may be insufficient. For many individuals, 28 days is not enough time to address deep-seated addiction issues. Long-term treatment or continued care post-discharge can be necessary for sustained recovery (Dennis M. L. et al., 2005). In this study, we implemented survival analysis techniques utilizing data gathered from initial assessments, including lifetime histories of substance use and treatment and follow-up interview information. These analyses were aimed at determining the duration between an individual's initial substance use and their first treatment, leading up to either 12 months of abstinence or their demise. In cases where individuals were still undergoing treatment, actively using substances, or had passed away by the last follow-up, these were considered right-censored in our analysis.

Observations over three years post-intake revealed that approximately 47% of individuals achieved a minimum of 12 months of

[227] Kelly, J. F., & Yeterian, J. D. (2011). The role of mutual-help groups in extending the framework of treatment. *Alcohol Research & Health*, 33(4), 350–355.

[228] Polcin, D. L., & Henderson, D. (2008). A clean and sober place to live: Philosophy, structure, and purported therapeutic factors in sober living houses. *Journal of Psychoactive Drugs*, 40(2), 153–159. https://doi.org/10.1080/02791072.2008.10400629

[229] McLellan, A. T., et al. (2005). Drug Dependence, a Chronic Medical Illness: Implications for Treatment, Insurance, and Outcomes Evaluation. *JAMA*, 284(13), 1689–1695. https://doi.org/10.1001/jama.284.13.1689

sobriety. The median duration from the initial substance use to complete cessation was recorded at 27 years. Furthermore, the median interval from the first engagement in treatment to the final usage instance spanned nine years. Notably, the journey to recovery was significantly prolonged in specific demographics, including males, individuals who initiated substance use before the age of 21—especially those starting before 15 years of age—as well as those who had undergone treatment on three or more occasions, and individuals experiencing high levels of mental distress.

These preliminary findings suggest a pattern wherein multiple care episodes spread over several years are commonplace in the recovery process. Instead of viewing these repeated episodes as a "cumulative dosage" of treatment, they might be more accurately perceived as indicative of the chronic nature of substance abuse. This perspective underscores the necessity for developing and assessing models focused on extended-term recovery management. This approach recognizes recovery's prolonged and often recurrent nature, emphasizing the need for sustained support and intervention strategies beyond traditional short-term treatment models.[230]

There are high costs and accessibility issues in the 28-day addiction treatment model. These programs can be expensive and inaccessible to everyone, especially those lacking insurance or adequate financial resources (McKay, J. R., 2009).[231]

Despite initial success, there are concerns about high relapse rates post-treatment. This raises questions about the effectiveness of the 28-day model in ensuring long-term sobriety (Simpson, D. D., & Joe, G. W., 2004).[232]

While the 28-day addiction treatment model has been a traditional approach with several benefits, including structure and a focus on abstinence, it faces criticism for its one-size-fits-all approach and

---

[230] Dennis, M.L., Scott, C.K., Funk, R., Foss, M.A. (2005) The duration and correlates of addiction and treatment careers. Retrieved from https://pubmed.ncbi.nlm.nih.gov/15797639/

[231] Ibid. McKay (2009). 131-135.

[232] Ibid. Simpson & Joe, (2004).

potential insufficiency in duration. Adaptability and continued care are vital aspects that need more emphasis in this model.

Addiction Recovery Rates

Recent studies in the field of addiction treatment reveal that the typical 28-day addiction treatment program yields a recovery success rate of around 20% (NIDA, 2020).[233]

This statistic underscores the initial effectiveness of such programs in addressing substance use disorders. Further, the research indicates a cumulative effect of treatment participation: with each additional treatment cycle, the likelihood of successful recovery increases by a comparable margin of 20% (McLellan et al., 2000). This suggests a progressive enhancement in treatment outcomes with repeated interventions.[234]

Moreover, ongoing support and encouragement in the recovery journey are pivotal. Individuals who consistently receive motivational and emotional support exhibit a higher propensity for sustained recovery, accentuating the importance of a supportive network in reinforcing treatment gains (Melemis, 2015). This points to the interplay of treatment participation and external support systems in enhancing long-term recovery prospects.[235]

A study by Eddy (1992) found that compliance with court-ordered substance abuse treatment among substance-abusing parents is as low as 20%. This indicates that while legal consequences can motivate some addicts, many may require additional interventions to engage in recovery effectively.[236]

---

[233] National Institute on Drug Abuse. (2020). Principles of Drug Addiction Treatment: A Research-Based Guide (Third Edition). Retrieved from https://www.drugabuse.gov/publications/principles-drug-addiction-treatment-research-based-guide-third-edition.
[234] McLellan, A. T., Lewis, D. C., O'Brien, C. P., & Kleber, H. D. (2000). Drug dependence, a chronic medical illness: Implications for treatment, insurance, and outcomes evaluation. *Journal of the American Medical Association, 284*(13), 1689-1695.
[235] Melemis, S. M. (2015). Relapse Prevention and the Five Rules of Recovery. *Yale Journal of Biology and Medicine, 88*(3), 325–332.
[236] Eddy, W. (1992). Motivating substance abusing parents in dependency court. *Juvenile and Family Court Journal, 43*, 11-19. Eddy (1992).

Literature on drug treatment efficacy consistently shows a disappointing 10 to 20% recovery rate, as highlighted by Copemann (1975). This suggests that traditional approaches to addiction treatment may not be sufficiently practical for a majority of individuals.[237]

A study focusing on opioid addiction by Hser et al. (2015) found that the long-term recovery rate for opioid addicts is low, with less than 30% achieving stable abstinence after 10-30 years of observation.[238]

Delos Reyes (2002) discusses the gap between the need for addiction treatment and the actual number of individuals receiving it, noting that less than 25% of those who could benefit from treatment receive it. The paper also highlights the effectiveness of even brief interventions in addiction treatment.[239]

Jones et al. (2009) surveyed drug and alcohol counselors recovering from addictions and found an overall relapse rate of approximately 38%. This highlights the challenges faced even by those knowledgeable about addiction.[240]

The efficacy of addiction treatment programs, particularly those of a 28-day duration, is marked by an initial 20% recovery rate. This rate is subject to improvement with each subsequent treatment cycle. The integration of continuous support and encouragement is crucial in bolstering these outcomes, highlighting the necessity of a holistic approach to addiction recovery. This underscores the complexity and chronic nature of addiction and the need for more effective and individualized treatment approaches.

---

[237] Copemann, C. D. (1975). Drug addiction: I. A theoretical framework for behavior therapy. *Psychological Reports, 37*, 947-958. Copemann (1975).

[238] Hser, Y., Evans, E., Grella, C., Ling, W., & Anglin, D. (2015). Long-term course of opioid addiction. *Harvard Review of Psychiatry, 23*, 76–89. Hser et al. (2015).

[239] Delos Reyes, C. M. (2002). Overcoming pessimism about the treatment of addiction. *JAMA, 287 14*, 1857. Delos Reyes (2002).

[240] Jones, T., Sells, J., & Rehfuss, M. C. (2009). How wounded the healers? The prevalence of relapse among addiction counselors in recovery from alcohol and other drugs. *Alcoholism Treatment Quarterly, 27*, 389-408. Jones et al. (2009).

STRATEGIES FOR IMPROVEMENT

The traditional 28-day model, popularized mainly in the United States, is based on the Minnesota Model developed in the 1950s. This model is centered around the principles of Alcoholics Anonymous (AA) and includes a combination of detoxification, group therapy, and the promotion of abstinence. However, recent advancements in addiction science and psychology have brought forward alternative approaches that may offer greater efficacy for some individuals.

Alternative Approaches to the 28-Day Model

Long-Term Residential Treatment — Extended residential programs, often lasting from 3 to 12 months, provide a more immersive and prolonged approach. Evidence is mounting that longer treatments can be more effective, especially for severe cases of addiction (McKay, J. R. (2009).[241]

Outpatient Treatment Programs — These programs allow individuals to live at home and maintain routine daily activities while attending treatment sessions. A study by McKay et al. (2010) found that intensive outpatient treatments can be as effective as inpatient treatments for many individuals struggling with addiction.[242]

Medication-Assisted Treatment (MAT) — MAT combines behavioral therapy and medications to treat substance use disorders. Research has shown its effectiveness, particularly in opioid addiction treatment (Volkow et al., 2014).[243]

---

[241] McKay, J. R. (2009). Continuing care research: What we have learned and where we are going. Journal of Substance Abuse Treatment, 36(2), 131-145. doi:10.1016/j.jsat.2008.10.004.

[242] McKay, J. R., Van Horn, D. H., Oslin, D. W., Lynch, K. G., Ivey, M., Ward, K., ... & Coviello, D. M. (2010). A randomized trial of extended telephone-based continuing care for alcohol dependence: Within-treatment substance use outcomes. Journal of Consulting and Clinical Psychology, 78(6), 912-923. doi:10.1037/a0020700.

[243] Volkow, N. D., Frieden, T. R., Hyde, P. S., & Cha, S. S. (2014). Medication-assisted therapies — tackling the opioid-overdose epidemic. New England Journal of Medicine, 370(22), 2063-2066. doi:10.1056/NEJMp1402780.

Cognitive Behavioral Therapy (CBT) — CBT is a short-term, goal-oriented counseling treatment that takes a hands-on, practical approach to problem-solving. Studies show its effectiveness in changing negative thought patterns that contribute to substance abuse (Magill & Ray, 2009).[244]

Contingency Management (CM) — CM provides tangible rewards to reinforce positive behaviors such as abstinence. Numerous studies have indicated its efficacy, especially in treating stimulant use disorders (Petry & Martin, 2002).[245]

Mindfulness and Holistic Therapies — Practices like yoga and meditation have been increasingly integrated into treatment programs. They are shown to reduce stress, a critical factor in relapse (Khanna & Greeson, 2013).[246]

With an esteemed background as a clinical pastoral counselor and extensive experience spanning over three decades, particularly in addiction treatment, my insights into faith-based addiction treatment methodologies are helpful. The holistic approach I advocate, emphasizing the benefits of biblical meditation and prayer, is a significant aspect of this discussion.

Delving into the realm of faith-based addiction treatment, it is essential to acknowledge the many benefits it offers. This approach is not merely about addressing the physical, mental, and emotional aspects of addiction but also involves nurturing the spiritual well-being of individuals. Incorporating biblical meditation and prayer into treatment regimes provides a unique dimension of healing and recovery.

Biblical meditation, distinct from other forms of meditation, involves deep reflection and contemplation on the Scriptures. This

---

[244] Magill, M., & Ray, L. A. (2009). Cognitive-behavioral treatment with adult alcohol and illicit drug users: A meta-analysis of randomized controlled trials. Journal of Studies on Alcohol and Drugs, 70(4), 516-527. doi:10.15288/jsad.2009.70.516.

[245] (Petry, N. M., & Martin, B. (2002). Low-cost contingency management for treating cocaine- and opioid-abusing methadone patients. Journal of Consulting and Clinical Psychology, 70(2), 398-405. doi:10.1037/0022-006X.70.2.398).

[246] (Khanna, S., & Greeson, J. M. (2013). A narrative review of yoga and mindfulness as complementary therapies for addiction. Complementary Therapies in Medicine, 21(3), 244-252. doi:10.1016/j.ctim.2013.01.008).

practice can offer profound spiritual insights and foster a sense of peace and purpose, which are crucial for individuals battling addiction. It serves as a grounding tool, enabling individuals to connect with their faith meaningfully, and often provides guidance and comfort during challenging times.

Prayer, another cornerstone of faith-based addiction treatment, offers direct communication with the divine. It allows individuals to express their fears, hopes, and gratitude, creating a sense of belonging and support. Prayer can be a powerful mechanism for coping with stress and the challenges that arise during the recovery process. It can also foster a sense of community, especially in groups, reinforcing the belief that one is not alone in their journey.

Integrating these spiritual practices in addiction treatment aligns with the holistic approach of treating the individual's mind, body, and spirit. This approach recognizes that addiction is not just a physical or mental struggle but also a spiritual one. By addressing the spiritual aspect, faith-based treatment can offer a comprehensive pathway to recovery, which can be especially effective for individuals with strong religious beliefs.

Furthermore, research has indicated the positive effects of spirituality and religious practices in recovery. For example, a study published in the journal "Substance Abuse and Rehabilitation" highlighted that spirituality could play a significant role in enhancing recovery, improving mental health outcomes, and reducing the likelihood of relapse (Geppert et al., 2007).[247]

This emphasis on the benefits of biblical meditation and prayer as part of a holistic approach to addiction treatment is well-founded. These practices offer unique benefits that can significantly aid recovery, providing comfort, guidance, and a sense of community to those in need.

Biblical meditation is a profoundly enriching spiritual practice that offers a multitude of benefits for both the soul and mind. Unlike common perceptions of meditation that often align with Eastern

---

[247] Geppert, C., Bogenschutz, M. P., & Miller, W. R. (2007). Development of a bibliography on religion, spirituality and addictions. Drug and Alcohol Review, 26(4), 389-395. doi:10.1080/09595230701373829

spiritual traditions, biblical meditation is a distinct practice deeply rooted in Christian theology and tradition.

One of the primary advantages of biblical meditation is its capacity to foster a profound connection with God. Engaging with Scripture through meditation allows individuals to delve deeper into the word of God, enhancing their understanding and appreciation of biblical teachings. This practice often involves pondering and reflecting upon specific passages, enabling a more personalized and intimate interaction with the Scriptures. It's a process that encourages believers to internalize and contemplate the teachings of the Bible, leading to a deeper spiritual awareness and a stronger relationship with God.

Furthermore, biblical meditation contributes significantly to mental and emotional well-being. By focusing on God's word, individuals can experience peace and stability, particularly in times of stress or turmoil. This form of meditation provides a spiritual anchor, helping practitioners to navigate life's challenges with greater resilience and a sense of divine support. The reflective nature of this practice promotes mental clarity, reducing anxiety and fostering a state of calmness.

Additionally, biblical meditation aids in moral and ethical decision-making. Regular engagement with Scripture through meditation sharpens one's understanding of Christian values and principles. This heightened moral consciousness guides individuals in making choices that align with their faith, leading to a more fulfilling and purposeful life.

It is also worth noting that biblical meditation can enhance one's sense of community and belonging. By meditating on shared scriptures, believers can feel a deeper connection to their faith community, fostering a sense of unity and shared purpose. This communal aspect of biblical meditation strengthens bonds within the church, encouraging mutual support and understanding among its members.

In summary, biblical meditation is a multifaceted practice that deepens one's relationship with God, promotes mental and emotional well-being, aids in ethical decision-making, and strengthens community bonds. It's a discipline that enriches the individual and the wider Christian community, offering a path to greater spiritual, mental, and emotional fulfillment.

Community and Peer Support Programs — Peer support programs, including 12-step groups and other mutual help organizations, can provide ongoing support post-treatment. Studies suggest that continued engagement in these groups can significantly improve long-term recovery outcomes (Kelly & Yeterian, 2011).[248]

Instead of treating the addict by giving them easier access to substances and behaviors of abuse, it's time the government recognizes addiction as a World War with the chances of human destruction. It's time governments fund addiction treatment similarly to their military.

The purpose of the military can be broadly understood through its primary roles and responsibilities, which are diverse and vary depending on the nation and its specific geopolitical context. Some of the military's essential functions are national defense, deterrence, peacekeeping, humanitarian assistance and relief, promotion of national interests, and internal security.

Can you see the parallel with the treatment of addictions?

The symbolic parallel between military strategies and the treatment of drug and behavioral addictions is an intriguing area to explore. Although distinct in their primary objectives, both realms share commonalities in their approach toward discipline, structure, and strategies for overcoming challenges.

In the military, discipline and structure are paramount. Soldiers are trained to follow orders, adhere to strict schedules, and maintain high standards of conduct. Similarly, in treating addictions, discipline is a critical component. Treatment programs often involve a structured environment where patients are expected to follow a routine, participate in scheduled therapy sessions, and adhere to rules that promote recovery (McKay, J. R., 2009). This structure provides a framework within which individuals can work towards overcoming their addictions.[249]

Military strategies often involve detailed planning, surveillance, and adapting to changing conditions on the battlefield. In addiction

---

[248] (Kelly, J. F., & Yeterian, J. D. (2011). The role of mutual-help groups in extending the framework of treatment. Alcohol Research & Health, 33(4), 350-355).

[249] McKay, J. R. (2009). Treating Substance Use Disorders with Adaptive Continuing Care. American Psychological Association. https://doi.org/10.1037/11882-000.

treatment, a similar approach is seen where treatment plans are personalized, and continuous monitoring is essential. Therapists and clinicians assess the patient's progress and modify treatment strategies based on their evolving needs (Simpson, D. D., & Joe, G. W., 2004).[250]

The military operates on teamwork, where soldiers rely on each other for support, motivation, and accomplishing missions. In addiction recovery, the support system, including group therapy, family involvement, and peer support, plays a crucial role. This support network provides encouragement, accountability, and a sense of community, essential for recovery (Kelly, J. F., & Greene, M. C., 2020).[251]

Military training prepares soldiers for various scenarios they might encounter. Similarly, in addiction treatment, individuals are equipped with coping skills and relapse prevention strategies. This preparation helps them to deal with potential triggers and challenges post-treatment, akin to a soldier being prepared for unexpected challenges in the field (Marlatt & Donovan, 2005).[252]

The military continually evaluates and improves strategies and tactics based on past experiences and emerging threats. Continuous evaluation is also crucial in addiction treatment. Treatment effectiveness is assessed, and programs are modified based on research and clinical outcomes, ensuring the approaches remain practical and relevant (Miller, W. R., & Rollnick, S., 2013).[253]

The parallels between military strategies and the treatment of drug and behavioral addictions are evident in their shared emphasis on discipline, structured approaches, adaptive strategies, teamwork, preparedness, and continuous improvement. These similarities

[250] Simpson, D. D., & Joe, G. W. (2004). A longitudinal evaluation of treatment engagement and recovery stages. Journal of Substance Abuse Treatment, 27(2), 89-97. https://doi.org/10.1016/j.jsat.2004.06.001.

[251] Kelly, J. F., & Greene, M. C. (2020). Addiction Recovery and Support Systems. In: Addiction Medicine: Science and Practice. Springer, Cham. https://doi.org/10.1007/978-3-319-63040-3_53-1.

[252] Marlatt, G. A., & Donovan, D. M. (Eds.). (2005). Relapse Prevention: Maintenance Strategies in the Treatment of Addictive Behaviors. Guilford Press.

[253] Miller, W. R., & Rollnick, S. (2013). Motivational Interviewing: Helping People Change (3rd ed.). Guilford Press.

underscore the importance of a well-structured and adaptive approach in both fields, highlighting how methodologies in one area can inform and enhance practices in another.

Bringing us home in the journey of unmasking addiction, the conventional 28-day model for addiction treatment, though beneficial in certain aspects, evidently falls short in addressing a topic that is intricate and composed of numerous aspects and the individualized nature of addiction recovery. It is increasingly apparent that the concept of a universal solution for addiction treatment is fundamentally flawed. The necessity for tailor-made treatment plans to accommodate each individual's unique requirements and situations cannot be overstated. Such plans should encompass diverse therapeutic—healing approaches and interventions that align with the patient's experiences and challenges.

Furthermore, integrating these varied treatment modalities demands robust support at the governmental level. This support is not limited to mere endorsement. Still, it extends to allocating resources, policy formulation, and implementation conducive to a more personalized and effective addiction treatment paradigm. In essence, a shift towards a more individualized and well-supported treatment framework is not only desirable but imperative for the advancement of addiction treatment methodologies.

The pivotal role of individualized care in addiction treatment is well-documented in numerous studies. For instance, a study published in the Journal of Substance Abuse Treatment highlights the enhanced effectiveness of personalized treatment plans over-generalized models (Journal of Substance Abuse Treatment, 45(1), 44-50). Additionally, the importance of governmental support in advancing addiction treatment strategies is echoed in a report by the Substance Abuse and Mental Health Services Administration, which underscores the critical need for policy and resource allocation to improve treatment outcomes (SAMHSA Publication No. PEP19-PL-Guide).[254] [255]

---

[254] Journal of Substance Abuse Treatment, 45(1), 44-50. https://store.samhsa.gov/sites/default/files/sma15-4131.pdf.

[255] SAMHSA Publication No. PEP19-PL-Guide. https://store.samhsa.gov/sites/default/files/substance-misuse-prevention-young-adults-pep19-pl-guide-1.pdf

The extensive range of addiction research cited in this publication underscores the necessity for a treatment paradigm that is general and centered around the individual, bolstered by robust government support. Such an approach not only acknowledges the unique requirements of those battling addiction but is also in harmony with the optimal strategies endorsed by foremost authorities in the domain. This perspective champions the idea that personalized care, informed by a broad spectrum of studies and expert opinions, is essential for addressing the multifaceted nature of addiction. It advocates for policies and programs that are flexible enough to adapt to each person's circumstances while still being grounded in the evidence-based practices identified through rigorous research. Doing so positions itself at the intersection of compassion and scientific excellence, aiming to provide the most effective and respectful care possible for individuals facing addiction challenges.

Conclusion: Unmasking Addiction

As we conclude our book, "Unmasking Addiction," it's crucial to reflect on the journey we've embarked upon together through a detailed exploration of six essential areas—spanning the spirit, soul, and body—this series aimed to shed light on the dimensional nature of addiction. We delved into the Spiritual and Behavioral Origins of the Addictive Process, explored the concept of the Addictive Personality, analyzed the interplay between Drugs and the Brain, and finally, navigated the pathways to Recovery and the challenges of Relapse. Our exploration was not just an academic exercise but a voyage toward understanding, compassion, and actionable knowledge.

By Unmasking the Spiritual Origins of the Addictive Process, we worked toward recognizing addiction's spiritual dimensions, which allows us to comprehend its profound impact on the human spirit. This understanding encourages a holistic approach to healing that integrates spiritual care with traditional therapeutic modalities (Miller, W. R., 1998).[256]

---

[256] Miller, W. R. (1998). Researching the spiritual dimensions of alcohol and other drug problems. Addiction, 93(7), 979–990. https://doi.org/10.1046/j.1360-0443.1998.9379793.x

By Unmasking the Behavioral Origins of the Addictive Process, we examined the behavioral patterns that contribute to addiction. We gained insights into how habits form and can be reshaped towards healthier alternatives (Duhigg, C., 2012).[257]

By Unmasking the Addictive Personality, we learned the concept of an addictive personality remains controversial, yet understanding the traits that predispose individuals to addiction can be invaluable in developing preventive and therapeutic strategies (Sussman, S., Lisha, N., & Griffiths, M., 2011).[258]

By Unmasking Drugs and the Brain, we journeyed through a scientific exploration into how substances hijack the brain's reward system, providing crucial insights into the biological underpinnings of addiction. This knowledge is essential for developing practical treatment approaches (Volkow, N. D., & Morales, M., 2015).[259]

By Unmasking Recovery, we learned recovery is a personal and dynamic journey that encompasses much more than abstinence. It involves the restoration of the mind, body, and spirit. Highlighting the diversity of recovery experiences encourages a more compassionate and individualized approach to healing (White, W. L., 2007).[260]

By Unmasking Relapse, we understood relapse as a part of the recovery process rather than a failure. This perspective shift allows for a more supportive and effective response to those in recovery. This perspective shift is crucial for individuals and their support networks (Marlatt, G. A., & Donovan, D. M. (Eds.)., 2005).[261]

In conclusion, "Unmasking Addiction" is a book dedicated

---

[257] Duhigg, C. (2012). The power of habit: Why we do what we do in life and business. Random House.

[258] Sussman, S., Lisha, N., & Griffiths, M. (2011). Prevalence of the Addictions: A Problem of the Majority or the Minority? Evaluation & the Health Professions, 34(1), 3–56. https://doi.org/10.1177/0163278710380124.

[259] Volkow, N. D., & Morales, M. (2015). The Brain on Drugs: From Reward to Addiction. Cell, 162(4), 712–725. https://doi.org/10.1016/j.cell.2015.07.046.

[260] White, W. L. (2007). Addiction recovery: Its definition and conceptual boundaries. Journal of Substance Abuse Treatment, 33(3), 229–241. https://doi.org/10.1016/j.jsat.2007.04.015.

[261] Marlatt, G. A., & Donovan, D. M. (Eds.). (2005). Relapse prevention: Maintenance strategies in the treatment of addictive behaviors. Guilford Press.

to comprehensively uncovering the complexities of addiction. By examining the interplay between the spirit, soul, and body in the addictive process, this series aimed to foster a deeper understanding of addiction's multifaceted nature. We hope the insights shared here will serve as a valuable resource for those seeking to understand more about addiction, whether for personal growth, to support a loved one, or to enhance professional practice in addiction counseling and recovery.

As we move forward, let us carry with us the knowledge that addiction is not merely a series of unfortunate choices or a fixed state of being but a treatable condition that encompasses the entire human experience. We can truly make a difference in the lives of those affected by addiction through compassion, understanding, and a willingness to explore beyond the surface.

BIBLE REFERENCES